NEW GENDER MAINSTREAMING SERIES ON DEVEL

Gender Mainstreaming in the Health Sector

Experiences in Commonwealth Countries

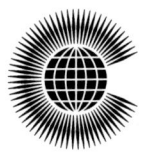

Commonwealth Secretariat

Commonwealth Secretariat
Marlborough House
Pall Mall, London SW1Y 5HX
United Kingdom

Published by the Commonwealth
Secretariat

Design: Wayzgoose
Cover design: Tony Leonard
Cover photograph:
Nancy Durrell McKenna
Printed in the United Kingdom
by Formara

Wherever possible, the
Commonwealth Secretariat uses
paper sourced from sustainable
forests or from sources that
minimise a destructive impact
on the environment.

Copies of this publication can
be ordered direct from:
The Publications Manager
Communications and Public
Affairs Division
Commonwealth Secretariat
Marlborough House
Pall Mall
London SW1Y 5HX
United Kingdom
Tel: +44 (0)20 7747 6342
Fax: +44 (0)20 7839 9081
E-mail:
r.jones-parry@commonwealth.int

Price: £8.99
ISBN: 0-85092-733-1

Web site:

http://www.thecommonwealth.org

Gender Management System Series:

Gender Management System Handbook

Using Gender Sensitive Indicators: A Reference Manual for Governments
and Other Stakeholders

Gender Mainstreaming in Agriculture and Rural Development: A Reference
Manual for Governments and Other Stakeholders

Gender Mainstreaming in Development Planning: A Reference Manual for
Governments and Other Stakeholders

Gender Mainstreaming in Education: A Reference Manual for Governments
and Other Stakeholders

Gender Mainstreaming in Finance: A Reference Manual for Governments
and Other Stakeholders

Gender Mainstreaming in Information and Communications: A Reference
Manual for Governments and Other Stakeholders

Gender Mainstreaming in Legal and Constitutional Affairs: A Reference
Manual for Governments and Other Stakeholders

Gender Mainstreaming in the Public Service: A Reference Manual for
Governments and Other Stakeholders

Gender Mainstreaming in Science and Technology: A Reference Manual for
Governments and Other Stakeholders

Gender Mainstreaming in Trade and Industry: A Reference Manual for
Governments and Other Stakeholders

Gender Mainstreaming in HIV/AIDS: Taking a Multisectoral Approach

A Quick Guide to the Gender Management System

A Quick Guide to Using Gender Sensitive Indicators

A Quick Guide to Gender Mainstreaming in Development Planning

A Quick Guide to Gender Mainstreaming in Education

A Quick Guide to Gender Mainstreaming in Finance

A Quick Guide to Gender Mainstreaming in the Public Service

A Quick Guide to Gender Mainstreaming in Trade and Industry

Contents

Preface

When Commonwealth Heads of Government adopted the Commonwealth Plan of Action on Gender and Development and its gender mainstreaming approach, the Gender and Youth Affairs Division of the Commonwealth Secretariat developed the concept of the Gender Management System (GMS) as a strategy for ensuring that a gender perspective is integrated into all government policies, planning and programmes. The GMS provides a network of structures, mechanisms and processes for achieving gender integration in different fields and it was felt that the health sector would benefit from the application of GMS principles. In response, the Health Department of the Commonwealth Secretariat embarked on the process of developing this manual on mainstreaming gender in the health sector.

A process of consultation and collaboration has been central to the development of the manual. Through a series of workshops in different regions of the Commonwealth, consensus was built up on the most effective way of applying the Gender Management System principles and methodology to the health sector. We capitalised on the flexibility of the GMS and were therefore able to take into account the different contexts prevailing in countries and the range of financial, human and other resources. The experiences gained from some countries have added a welcome practical dimension which we hope will assist other countries to adapt the approach to their own particular circumstances.

This manual has been produced to provide support and guidance to policy-makers, planners, non-governmental organisations, institutions and staff working in the health sector. The expectation is that it will increase gender mainstreaming and also encourage partnerships between all providers and recipients of health services in both public and private sectors as they all work towards increasing the effectiveness of the health sector for both women and men.

Acknowledgements

We thank all the participants, facilitators and resource persons who attended the workshops; their contributions have greatly enriched the manual.

We are also grateful to:

- All our member governments who hosted the workshops, and our partners who contributed resources to enable participants to attend;

- The Commonwealth Medical Association, joint organisers of the workshops;

- Ms Marianne Haslegrave, Dr Rawwida Baksh-Sooden, Dr Clement Chela and Mrs Janey Parris who contributed to the draft manual;

- Professor Stephen Matlin, former Director of the Human Resources Development Division, who conceptualised the manual;

- Dr Judith May Parker, former Deputy Director of the Gender and Youth Affairs Division.

The project was managed by Mrs Janey Parris, Chief Programme Officer, Health Department.

1. Mainstreaming Gender in the Health Sector: An Overview

Gender Inequality and Women's Health

In the twentieth century significant advances were made in raising the status of women. Prior to that, women faced discrimination in the political, legal, economic, social and other spheres of life. In many countries women, unlike men, did not have the right to vote nor did they enjoy basic human rights. They were clearly in a disadvantaged position in comparison to men. Gradually, progress was made in some countries and women began to enjoy some rights such as recognition of their independent legal status and the right to inherit and dispose of property. In employment, not only was it acknowledged that women had the right to all types and levels of work but it was also accepted that they had the right to equal pay for work of equal value. Many countries recognised that women had the right of access to all levels of education and should be given the opportunity to participate in all disciplines and reach the highest educational and professional levels. Slowly, women gained more access to political power and decision-making positions. A major advance was the recognition of good health as a fundamental human right for women and men that should be promoted and protected. It was also accepted that women had a right to full and equal access to all health services and that their special needs should be taken into account in providing these services. There was increasing awareness that women should have control of what happens to their bodies.

In spite of these advances, the overriding picture, especially in less developed countries and among poor and marginalised people everywhere, was of persistent discrimination against women in all aspects of life. Even where women's rights had been incorporated into international law or national legislation and policy, the reality was that, at national level, implementation was slow. In their daily lives women still did not enjoy their rights. While it was true that many men were also

. . . the overriding picture, especially in less developed countries and among poor and marginalised people everywhere, was of persistent discrimination against women in all aspects of life.

If women are to gain better access to health services, they must be given the opportunity to work in partnership with men at all levels of the health sector.

denied full enjoyment of their rights, it was very apparent that there was a large gap between women and men, with women being overwhelmingly at a disadvantage.

Improvement in health status remains a challenge for both women and men. However, the problem is more acute for women. There is a disparity between women and men in their ability to gain access to appropriate health care. The low health status of women in less developed countries has been identified as a major obstacle to development. Yet action to promote women's health remains inadequate.

If women are to gain better access to health services, they must be given the opportunity to work in partnership with men at all levels of the health sector, including the highest levels of policy-making. Together they must ensure that women's specific needs are identified and addressed in the manner that is most appropriate for them.

Moving from Women and Health to Gender and Health

Since the 1950s, there have been progressive changes in the way in which women are perceived in development planning. Caroline Moser, in *Gender Planning and Development: Theory, Practice and Training*, observed that prior to the International Women's Year Conference, held in Mexico in 1975, the approach taken to women's role in development was based on a social welfare concept. Consequently, as far as providing health care for women was concerned, the focus was on areas such as maternal and child health, nutrition and hygiene. There was a shift in perception when the International Women's Year Conference stated quite clearly that women were major, though unrecognised, contributors to the development process. This led to the emergence of the concept of 'Women in Development' (WID). Gradually, emphasis shifted to the 'poverty', 'equity', and 'efficiency' approaches until the 1990s when the focus was on the 'empowerment' and 'integration' approaches.

Table 1. Evolution of Approaches from Women in Development to Gender and Development

Period	Approach	Characteristics
1950s–1970s	Welfare approach	Linked to the social welfare model. Focused on women's practical needs: maternal and child health, nutrition, hygiene, education, food distribution programmes.
1970s	Poverty approach	Perceived issue as underdevelopment, rather than gender subordination. Aimed to improve material conditions of women's lives, enabling them to catch up with men through income generation, skills training, and access to marketing and credit.
1975–1985 UN Decade for Women	Equity approach	Concentrated on women's strategic needs, advocating changes in the economic, legal, social and ideological realities of women's situation. Equity projects encompassed consciousness-raising initiatives, as well as practical action in areas such as legal rights and access to credit.
1990s	Efficiency approach	Harnessed women's labour to make development more efficient. Assumed that women's increased economic participation would lead to increased equity.
1990s	Empowerment approach	Focus on strategic needs as identified by women. Concentrated on changing practices and enabling people to define their own agenda, rather than on changing laws, rules or frameworks.
1990s	Integration approach	Recognises that society assigns different gender roles to women and men. Stresses the need for both women and men to have access to and control over resources and decision-making processes. Integrates gender awareness and competence into 'mainstream' development.

At the international level, the achievement of gender equality has been regarded as a matter for priority action. Resolutions, declarations and conventions agreed at various world conferences and summit meetings in the twentieth century enshrined women's rights in general, with some paying specific attention to women's health rights. Table 2 provides an outline of some of these meetings and highlights some relevant outcomes.

Table 2. International Landmarks in Women's Equality

Date	Meeting/event	Relevant outcomes
1949	UN Universal Declaration of Human Rights	Asserted that everyone should enjoy fundamental human rights.
1975	International Women's Year Conference	Asserted that there should be equality of rights for women and initiated a Decade of Action to achieve goals of equality between women and men.
1975–1985	UN Decade for Women	Action to improve women's economic, political, legal and social circumstances.
1979	UN Convention on the Elimination of All Forms of Discrimination Against Women (CEDAW)	Affirmed women's equal rights in all areas of life and set up a Committee to which all governments that had ratified the Convention should present periodic reports on implementation.
1985	UN End of Decade Conference, Nairobi	Nairobi Forward Looking Strategies set out further measures for implementing action to achieve equality for women. Governments agreed to set up National Women's Machineries.
1990	World Conference on the Rights of the Child	Included targeting of maternal health and reduction in maternal mortality through improved nutrition and health care.
1993	Vienna Declaration and Programme of Action	Recognised the human rights of women and girl-children as an inalienable, integral and indivisible part of universal human rights.
1994	International Conference on Population and Development, Cairo	Asserted rights of women to sexual and reproductive health.
1995	World Summit for Social Development, Copenhagen	Advocated the effective participation of women in development.
1995	UN Fourth World Conference on Women, Beijing	Agreed on the Beijing Declaration and Platform for Action. Identified Women and Health as one of the 12 critical areas for action. Asserted the right of women to the fullest enjoyment of health, including sexual and reproductive health, throughout their lives.
1995	Commonwealth Heads of Government Meeting, Auckland	Endorsed the Commonwealth Plan of Action on Gender and Development and urged governments to implement it.

Increasingly, the emphasis has moved away from a focus on sex discrimination, which is attributed to biological differences, to an understanding of how different roles assigned by society to women and men, i.e. gender roles, affect equality issues. The Gender and Development (GAD) approach recognises the profound effect which gender-based roles have on the sharing of responsibilities and access to resources and benefits between women and men. It also notes that these roles have a major impact on the balance of power between women and men to the disadvantage of women.

The GAD position is that these inequalities were created by society and must therefore be rectified by it. GAD advocates a change of attitude from viewing inequalities between women and men as 'women's issues' to a broader approach which states that inequalities arise out of gender roles and that they should therefore be of equal concern to both women and men. Instead of being marginalised, problems arising from these inequalities should be addressed as part of mainstream policies and programmes. This process, which is known as 'gender mainstreaming', is seen as the logical and fair way forward towards achieving gender equality and equity. GAD puts up a strong argument for the empowerment of women. It calls for a fundamental change of attitude, which should result in better-targeted policies and programmes to meet the needs of both women and men.

However, GAD goes beyond arguing for women's empowerment to state that there are areas in which men also have special needs. It raises awareness of the fact that the life courses of women and men are different because of the different roles which society assigns to them. Development policies do not have an identical impact on women and men because of these differences. In the GAD approach, the impact of gender roles becomes a factor in all analyses of data to be used for policy-making and programme planning. GAD also takes into account the changing nature of gender roles which differ according to historical time, location and the environment within which a particular society functions. This strengthens the case for continuously applying gender analysis to ensure that these changes are identified. The GAD approach involves a more comprehensive understanding of factors which hinder women from achieving equality. It highlights their status relative to the status of men and identifies women's special needs as a result of their lower status. From the GAD perspective, the achievement of gender equality is a task for the whole of society, women and men alike. As men become partners with women in the move towards gender equality, men themselves become beneficiaries of this process of change.

The 1995 Commonwealth Plan of Action adopted the GAD and gender mainstreaming approach. This is reflected in the Commonwealth Vision for Women.

. . . the life courses of women and men are different because of the different roles which society assigns to them.

The Commonwealth Vision for Women

The Commonwealth works towards a world in which women and men have equal rights and opportunities at all stages of their lives to express their creativity in all fields of human endeavour, and in which women are respected and valued as equal and able partners in establishing values of social justice, equity, democracy and respect for human rights. Within such a framework of values, women and men will work in collaboration and partnership to ensure people-centred sustainable development for all nations.

The *Commonwealth Plan of Action* identified women's health as one of its 15 critical areas for action. The Update to the Commonwealth Plan of Action on Gender and Development, *Advancing the Commonwealth Agenda for Gender Equality into the New Millennium, 2000–2005,* supported the gender mainstreaming approach and advocated its use in new and emerging social, economic and political changes occurring worldwide, all of which have major gender implications.

Policy-makers and practitioners in the health field are presented with a considerable challenge as they make the transition from WID to GAD. It is not simply a question of improving delivery of services to address women's health issues, for example maternal and child health, family planning and screening for breast and cervical cancer. Nor is it enough to move one step beyond this by also paying attention to services for men, for example screening for prostate cancer. Gender mainstreaming requires the health sector to identify, analyse and develop policies to end gender imbalances across the whole spectrum of health care. Gender mainstreaming also calls for the re-examination and elimination of many gender biases in the health field which are rooted in the culture and conditioning of society.

The following examples illustrate how gender biases can affect the provision of health care:

- Analysis of data from many developed countries shows that the diagnosis of heart disease in women often occurs at a later stage than in men and that treatment is less vigorous, with the result that prognosis is markedly poorer. The underlying reasons for women's higher mortality rates arise from a combination of factors: the use of diagnostic/symptomatic models that were based on research on men rather than women; misconceptions about the relative prevalence of heart disease that have falsely presented it as a 'male' disease; the development and optimisation of drug therapies based largely or exclusively on male patients; and different attitudes by the medical profession to treatment of the disease in men and women.

- On the other hand, there are instances where diseases are known to be equally common in men and women but where men are presenting at a more advanced stage for diagnosis and treatment, with an adverse impact on outcomes. This applies, for example, to diabetes and hypertension in the Caribbean. Analysis suggests that the root causes of this phenomenon include a culture that encourages a 'macho' self-image in men which inhibits admission of weakness or ill-health; unavailability of 'male-friendly' health services that are accessible at times and places that are convenient for men; and the absence of health education programmes in schools and the wider community to make men aware of the health risks they face and to encourage them to take responsibility for their health.

Practical Considerations in Gender Mainstreaming

As a follow-up to the twentieth century world conferences which asserted that women's rights were human rights and affirmed that women had a right to equality in all aspects of their lives, including health, governments agreed to adopt policies and programmes to enforce these rights. The challenge facing governments can be grasped by considering the following six factors which are vital elements in any comprehensive strategy to mainstream gender in the health sector:

a) Developing and implementing gender-sensitive policies;
b) Identifying priority areas for action;
c) Mobilising resources;

To achieve gender equality in any sector, including the health sector, it is necessary to have an 'enabling environment'.

d) Introducing National Women's Machineries
e) Involving men;
f) Taking a dynamic and flexible approach.

The following two critical issues which cut across the six factors that contribute to a gender mainstreaming strategy will also be considered:

- **Training:** Everyone involved in the process of gender mainstreaming in the health sector must have an understanding of what is meant by gender issues. This training should not be confined to a few experts but should be provided for all those involved, both providers and recipients of health services.

- **Health Information Systems:** It is important that information is collected on the health status of both women and men before gender mainstreaming is introduced. This will form the basis for making an assessment of the outcomes of the gender mainstreaming process. Doing this requires the setting up of an efficient and comprehensive health information system which relies on the collection and analysis of sex-disaggregated data, and continuous monitoring and evaluation. This information can then be used to plan health programmes which respond better to the different needs of people.

a) Developing and implementing gender-sensitive policies

To achieve gender equality in any sector, including the health sector, it is necessary to have an 'enabling environment'. This environment is created by the following inter-related factors:
- political will and administrative commitment
- international, regional and national mandates
- constitutional and legal framework.

Creating an enabling environment: political will and administrative commitment

This is a vital element in the development of an environment which is supportive of gender mainstreaming and the introduction of a Gender Management System. Evidence of political commitment can be seen in actions such as:

- The government signs or ratifies international and regional conventions and agreements for achieving gender equality. This can include international agreements such as the Beijing Declaration and Platform for Action. The government also devotes adequate administrative resources to ensure that the political will is translated into action.

- The government establishes National Women's Machineries (NWMs) with a mandate to promote gender equality and gives them a sufficiently high status to enable them to influence policy and decision-making in all sections of the public sector.

International, regional and national mandates

The government implements mandates given to achieve gender equality. For instance, the Beijing Declaration and Platform for Action provides a mandate for achieving gender equality in all areas of life, including the health sector.

The Beijing Declaration

We are convinced that women's empowerment and their full participation on the basis of equality in all spheres of society, including participation in the decision-making process and access to power are fundamental for the achievement of equality, development and peace.

We are convinced that the explicit recognition and reaffirmation of the right of all women to control all aspects of their health, in particular their own fertility, is basic to their empowerment.

The Beijing Platform for Action has five strategic objectives, which governments agreed to pursue to achieve the goal of gender equality in health:

- To increase women's access throughout the life cycle to appropriate, affordable and quality health care, information and related services;

- To strengthen preventive programmes that promote women's health;

Policies and programmes to achieve gender equality have a greater chance of success where the national constitution guarantees equality of women and men . . .

- To undertake gender-sensitive initiatives that address sexually-transmitted diseases, HIV/AIDS, and sexual and reproductive health issues;

- To promote research and disseminate information on women's health;

- To increase resources and monitor follow-up for women's health.

Constitutional and legal framework

Policies and programmes to achieve gender equality have a greater chance of success where the national constitution guarantees equality of women and men and prohibits discrimination on the basis of sex. A supportive environment is also created when there are existing laws, or new laws are enacted or legal reform is undertaken to end gender-based discrimination. The legislation should be comprehensive, covering all aspects of life, for example nationality, marriage, custody of children, inheritance, ownership of property, including land, and credit. Barbados provides a good example of how a government can carry out reforms to provide a supportive legislative framework. In 1978 the National Commission on the Status of Women identified 212 areas in which women faced discrimination. By 1998 95 per cent of the necessary action had been taken to remove these discriminatory practices.

The value of having a supportive constitutional and legislative framework for gender mainstreaming is summed up in the *Gender Management System Handbook* as follows:

This legitimises the efforts of social partners working towards gender equality and equity, and also creates a mechanism for corporate, state and individual accountability. The legal framework establishes a rights perspective and renders women as claimants rather than as beneficiaries. It sets standards and delineates categories of people or institutions that are obligated to fulfill these rights and entitlements. It enables women to negotiate their rights at the personal and societal levels.

In many countries the enabling environment is weak and one of the tasks of the National Women's Machineries and civil society organisations concerned with gender equality issues is to lobby for weak elements to be strengthened. Many governments have made only piecemeal attempts at implementing policies and programmes to achieve gender equality. Although Commonwealth governments have carried out legislative reform, introduced new legislation and issued policy statements supporting gender equality, often a visible gap remains between policy and practice, and between rhetoric and reality. National Women's Machineries are accorded a low status and continue to be under-resourced; often the expectation is that responsibility for achieving gender equality rests with them. The Commonwealth Secretary-General's report of 1999 on the implementation of the Commonwealth Plan of Action on Gender and Development, *Learning By Sharing*, highlighted weaknesses in National Women's Machineries which reflect the gaps in the enabling environment:

Over 50 per cent of National Women's Machineries are still placed within traditional sector ministries such as social development, family welfare, health, national heritage and culture, which are wrongly perceived as 'women's issues'. Many are subsumed under other departments which are given greater priority within these ministries.

Commenting on resources for National Women's Machineries, the report stated:

There has been no improvement in this area since 1996. In 1999, all but six countries have had some constraints placed on their capacity and ability to implement the national women/gender policy and programme to the Year 2000.

It is therefore very encouraging when political commitment is apparent. Namibian participants attending a Commonwealth workshop on Gender Management Systems in the Health Sector commented:

Namibia's greatest strength is seen to be the political commitment of the State which provides a rallying ground for gender equality and equal representation at all levels and in all sectors of society. The establishment of the Gender Co-ordinating Body in the Office of the President, the setting up of a Women and Child Abuse centre, and Adolescent Multi-purpose Centres to be used by both girls and boys are evidence of movement in the right direction.

Some Commonwealth countries have introduced initiatives which have enhanced the status of women in the health sector,

Many governments have made only piecemeal attempts at implementing policies and programmes to achieve gender equality.

Health providers do not usually focus on gender equality as a special issue in the planning and delivery of health care.

for example reviewing and raising the status of women as health workers; addressing the reproductive health needs of women; and responding to gender-based needs in the ageing process. However, attempts to achieve gender equality in health have been limited and only partially successful.

On the whole, the cycle of change which moves from adopting gender-sensitive policies and language to developing attitudes which accept gender equality and then actually changing to behaviour which clearly demonstrates gender equality, has not been completed. In many cases, the transition from one stage to the next has been slow or has not materialised.

Instead, they tend to limit themselves to targeting special groups such as women and children. The assumption is that all other health services are equally accessible to both women and men and that they benefit equally from them. This is often not the case. Health providers do not usually focus on gender equality as a special issue in the planning and delivery of health care. Where data have been collected, they point to one sex, usually women, being disadvantaged in access to, or in quality of, treatment. This can be caused by lack of resources as, for instance, when women do not have adequate money, transport or time to reach health care facilities. Poor access can also be the consequence of societal customs. For example, women may not be allowed to seek medical attention on their own but have to be accompanied by a male relative, or they may only be allowed to seek treatment from a woman doctor. Designers and providers of health care may also unwittingly limit women's access because they do not fully understand or respect their needs. This can happen if the health programme is so focused on specific goals such as safe motherhood, screening for cervical and breast cancer, or child immunisation, that other services, some of which might meet the special needs of women, are neglected. Similarly, services which are only available during working hours may limit accessibility for working men.

Commitment by administrators is vital for achieving gender equality in health. This is particularly so because the provision of good health care depends on services provided by government ministries and agencies which are outside the health ministry. Ministries, departments and agencies responsible for finance, planning, the environment, food and water supply, safety, waste management and transport all deal with services which impact on the health of the population. For successful gender mainstreaming in the health sector, it is imperative that in addition to the Ministry of Health and its related agencies, other ministries, departments and agencies whose activities help determine the quality of health enjoyed by the population, should be part of a national health action plan. This complex plan would require significant administrative commitment from all involved. Political will at the highest level of government will be essential to ensure a high level of administrative commitment.

Effective gender mainstreaming in health is dependent on increased gender awareness and sensitivity at all levels of society. Appropriate training for different groups of stakeholders is therefore essential. Policy-makers and practitioners must develop the capacity to analyse policies, plans and service delivery from a gender perspective, using sex-disaggregated data and taking into account the differential impact which policies and programmes could have on the health of women and men. The general public who will be beneficiaries, carers or partners in preventive health care programmes should also receive education information. This can be done through health information programmes, media campaigns and any other informal opportunities for education which exist in a particular environment.

Two critical gaps in the enabling environment which impede progress in gender mainstreaming in health were identified by participants at Commonwealth workshops:

- **A gap between policy-making and implementation.**
  Even strong policy statements supporting gender mainstreaming in health are not necessarily followed by implementation.

- **A gap between gender awareness and attitudes.**
  Even when training and information campaigns have raised the level of gender awareness, this has often remained an academic exercise which has not led to the required change in attitude and behaviour.

Effective gender mainstreaming in health is dependent on increased gender awareness and sensitivity at all levels of society.

*Research must
. . . have a special
objective to reach
out to all groups
in the community
in order to find
out about their
real needs . . .*

b) Identifying priority areas

In order to identify priority areas for action in health care it is first of all necessary to carry out a comprehensive review of all sectors of the existing health-care system. Existing mechanisms for determining health priorities which do not incorporate a gender perspective are generally unsatisfactory. All too often the database on which decisions about priorities are made is inadequate. There is, therefore, recourse to identifying priorities on the basis of international campaigns or local estimates, rather than on accurate, comprehensive and up-to-date data. This situation can only be rectified by the setting up of an efficient health information system which can collect, analyse and interpret sex-disaggregated data and disseminate the information so that it can be used in planning processes.

The development of a more complete and accurate picture requires research which goes beyond the problems with which patients present at hospitals, clinics and other health facilities. There are well-documented experiences from many countries of women and girls who are too frightened to report health problems because they are caused by violence and abuse perpetrated against them in the home or outside. In other regions, where the culture expects adolescents to be 'silent' about their needs, it is similarly difficult to ascertain their real needs. Research must, therefore, have a special objective to reach out to all groups in the community in order to find out about their real needs, including those which are not mentioned initially for various reasons. The research must be sufficiently broad-based to identify gender-related health needs associated with issues such as poor nutrition, anaemia, sexual and reproductive health, early motherhood, sexually transmitted infections and HIV/AIDS. It should include responses from the widest possible range of groups, including target and focus groups, in the society.

Methods which have been used to implement programmes in certain priority areas have themselves contributed to perpetuating or even widening inequalities. Undoubtedly, Maternal and Child Health (MCH), Safe Motherhood and Mother and Baby programmes have all made significant contributions to the reduction of maternal and neo-natal mortality. However there are limitations in this approach. An over-rigorous focus on the health needs of women as they carry out their role as mothers inadvertently neglects the needs of adolescent girls or post-menopausal women. It may also lead to neglect of the priority health needs of men. To avoid this, it is advisable that in setting priorities there should be an awareness of people's changing needs as they go through their life cycle. Differences occur because of the stage of life, for example adolescence, middle age, post menopause and old age, and also because of gender-based roles. Recognising this, some governments have changed to more broad-based programmes, as reported by participants from Malaysia.

The Family Health Programme in Malaysia

Malaysia moved from a Maternal and Child Health Programme to a Family Health Programme designed to take on a life-span approach. The new programme therefore had the following ten areas of focus: maternal health, child health, school health, well-woman clinics, family planning clinics, care of the elderly, adolescent health, mental health, rehabilitation and the care of children with special needs.

Health issues which are gender-based may require special programmes. This may apply, for instance, to rape cases. Many women do not report rape because law enforcement and medical personnel are often insensitive in their response. It is not unusual for women to be subjected to lengthy, unsympathetic and embarrassing questioning and examination by the police and social workers. Only after going through that ordeal are they given treatment for their injuries. Not surprisingly, many women refuse to report rape incidents. Malaysia has therefore introduced One Stop Centres based in hospitals where survivors of domestic violence and sexual assault can receive sensitive treatment from a range of services.

c) Mobilising resources for gender mainstreaming

In many countries, governments are introducing wide-reaching and fundamental reforms to their health systems to improve their relevance, sustainability, efficiency and cost-effectiveness.

has been accompanied by the establishment of Ministries Responsible for Women's Affairs, Women's Bureaux/Departments and the designation of officers as Gender Focal Points in ministries. These mechanisms have had some success in encouraging the development and strengthening of National Gender/Women's Policies and Plans of Action. Some reporting, monitoring and evaluation processes have also been put in place.

Although National Women's Machineries have succeeded in making notable advances in the promotion of gender equality, they have clearly had many limitations. Often they have been located in a marginal ministry with little political clout and therefore they could not participate meaningfully in mainstream political and decision-making processes. Their impact has been limited because they lacked leadership and management capacity, human, financial and material resources, and training and linkages with key sectors in the public sector or with important stakeholders in NGOs and civil society. If National Women's Machineries are to fulfil their role effectively they must overcome these limitations. This can only be done through the commitment and support of governments. They must also make a transition from focusing on women's issues to looking at gender issues. As they move to the promotion of gender integration, they will need to win men's commitment to the process. They will also have to gain acceptance of gender issues in the mainstream of all analysis, policy formulation and programme implementation.

Such a refocusing of priorities will require National Women's Machineries to redefine their roles, responsibilities and strategies. An initial step has been taken by some National Women's Machineries which have changed their titles to Gender Affairs Ministries or Departments. Others have started to emphasise their role as catalytic change agents which influence government policy. Generally, National Women's Machineries recognise that they need to move away from leaving responsibility for promoting gender equality in the hands of a few individuals to sharing responsibility with a wider group in the public and private sectors.

e) Involving men

The achievement of gender equality involves a process of change. In any situation where change is required there is likely to be resistance from those who perceive that their interests are threatened. It is, therefore, not unexpected to find that many men, who regard the move towards gender equality in the health sector as a threat to their own status, resist such changes. The challenge is to educate and sensitise men to understand gender issues and accept that gender equality is part of women's human rights. It is equally important to convince men that gender equality in health will be beneficial not only to women but also to men.

Training in gender awareness does not automatically lead to a change in attitudes. As participants in a Commonwealth workshop on gender mainstreaming in the health sector commented:

There was increasing awareness of gender issues among males in the health sector which was heavily female-dominated, although the majority of nurses were women while the majority of doctors were men. Increase in gender awareness brought little response. Sensitisation workshops did not appear to have the desired effect on attitudes.

Clearly, to convince men it is essential to show them how they will benefit from gender equality. The GAD approach supports this position and recognises that, just like women, men also have particular health needs and problems. Experience indicates that convincing men that gender mainstreaming not only improves women's health care, but also leads to better health provision for men, is the most effective way of winning men's support. Examples from Belize, South Africa and the Caribbean show the types of health issues which are relevant to men and which can be used to convince them that gender mainstreaming is in their interest.

The challenge is to educate and sensitise men to understand gender issues and accept that gender equality is part of women's human rights.

> ## Acting against Domestic Violence in Belize
>
> In Belize it was demonstrated that men, as well as women, can benefit from legislation which is properly drafted from a gender perspective. Women are the main victims of domestic violence and therefore the main users of the Domestic Violence Act, which was passed in 1992. Yet since the Act became law, the numbers of men seeking assistance under the provision has been slowly increasing.

Some countries have tackled the problem of many health facilities not being 'male-friendly'. Health programmes have been geared towards women and children, excluding men from participation in many decisions which should really involve them. These countries have therefore sought active male involvement in family planning with a 'male motivation' campaign. In one instance, a maternal and child health programme was aimed at strengthening male responsibility in reproductive health issues, because initially men were left out of the information/communication process and probably also felt excluded from services which catered primarily for the needs of women and children.

> ## Using Gender Analysis in South Africa
>
> In South Africa, it was gender analysis that revealed inadequacies in the provision of health care for men. Provision had been made for free health care for women and for children under six years old. Men had been disadvantaged by limited access to health services. There was minimal, if any, male focus within the health system and negative attitudes towards males persisted among health workers.

Meeting Men's Health Needs in the Caribbean

Caribbean countries have also launched programmes to increase men's involvement. In Barbados, national awareness campaigns to promote screening and early detection of cancer included not only breast and cervical cancer, but also prostate cancer. In St Kitts and Nevis, the Family Planning Association organised conferences dealing specifically with issues relevant to men. Discussions in which the men took part ranged from sexual and reproductive health to domestic violence and the need for men to take responsibility for their own actions.

Men, no less than women, may suffer ill health as a result of ignorance, prejudice and the existence of 'taboos'. These factors either prevent people from seeking help or result in a health system that ignores their real needs. There is a wide range of anecdotal evidence to this effect in the Caribbean, as illustrated by the following:

- The reluctance of women to report domestic violence and sexual abuse and assault has complex determinants. What is very noticeable in the Caribbean is the role played by the attitudes of family members and society in general. Opinions are expressed about what the woman should tolerate and the perceived undesirable consequences if a woman loses her home and economic stability as a result of her prosecuting the man.

- High rates of obesity among women in the Caribbean have led to high levels of diabetes and cardiovascular disease. This reflects patterns of socialisation which have not sensitised women sufficiently to the links between physical exercise, healthy diets, lifestyle and good health.

- Caribbean men are significantly more reluctant to visit health clinics than women. This has been attributed to various reasons including 'macho behaviour' where men do not want to appear to be weak; the lack of 'male-friendly' services because many services have evolved from maternal and child health facilities; and failure to socialise men so that

There should also be a gender balance in all decision-making, professional and technical processes, for example policy-making, consultation, teaching and research.

they become used to using maternal and child care services in the same way that women do. Men therefore tend to put off seeking health care until they present at clinics with serious or advanced conditions. They are especially reluctant to seek diagnosis or treatment for conditions which are related to their sexual function. This accounts for their reluctance to access health facilities if they suspect that there will be a diagnosis of either diabetes or hypertension, both of which they associate with possible impotence.

The examples from the Caribbean are not unique to that region and constitute the type of problems faced when efforts are made to achieve gender equality in health care by removing disadvantages to men.

f) Taking a dynamic and flexible approach

Health systems need to be dynamic, flexible and innovative rather than static, so that they can respond adequately to changing health needs. As society undergoes economic, social, environmental, lifestyle, nutritional and other changes, national health systems have to be alert to the possible impact which these changes can have on people's health. Appropriate changes should be made in health care. In the same way, relevant changes should be introduced to ensure continuing responsiveness to gender-based needs. This can be done by setting up a framework within which each component of the health system has mechanisms through which the gender perspective becomes automatically visible. Such mechanisms must be comprehensive and must operate at all levels and in all sub-sectors; they must operate in primary, secondary and tertiary health care, and in both public and private health care facilities. There should also be a gender balance in all decision-making, professional and technical processes, for example policy-making, consultation, teaching and research. This gender perspective must be promoted through the collection of sex-disaggregated data and must be included in all monitoring and evaluation exercises.

Such changes will not be achieved instantly because they are processes which require time to be accepted, assimilated and implemented. As the health system is effecting these changes, sectors of government and society will also be under-going change due to other factors. It is, therefore, vital that the health system has the capacity to manage a fluid and changing environment which includes changing gender needs. A strong argument for mainstreaming gender into the health sector as a matter of urgency is the fact that nearly all Commonwealth countries are now engaged in very substantial reform of their health systems. This involves the introduction of major changes and also provides an opportune time for introducing gender mainstreaming as part of the whole process of change.

2. Gender and Health: Clarifying the Issues

Understanding the Concept of Gender Mainstreaming

An understanding of the concept of gender is essential if a management system for mainstreaming gender into the health sector is to be set up. Far too often gender is regarded as being identical to 'sex' or 'women's issues'. In reality, gender refers not just to women but to both women and men.

The following definitions explain how sex and gender are different yet inter-related.

Sex and gender

'Sex' identifies the biological differences between women and men. 'Gender' refers to the array of socially constructed roles, attitudes, behaviours and values which determine in large measure women's and men's differential access to resources, status, influence and power. Sex and gender are interactive, but whilst sex and its associated biological functions are programmed genetically, gender roles and power relations vary across cultures and through different times in human development and are thus amenable to change.

Gender

Gender can be defined as the set of characteristics, roles and behaviour patterns that distinguish women from men, which are constructed not biologically, but socially and culturally. The sex of an individual is biologically determined, whereas gender characteristics are socially constructed – a product of nurturing, conditioning, and socio-cultural norms and expectations. These characteristics change over time and from one culture to another. Gender also refers to the web of cultural symbols, normative concepts and internalised self-images, which, through a process of social construction, define masculine and feminine roles and articulate these roles within power relationships.

Source: *Gender Management System Handbook*, Commonwealth Secretariat

Gender mainstreaming, which is the approach taken in setting up a Gender Management System in the health sector, has been defined in the *Gender Management System Handbook* as follows:

Gender Mainstreaming

This term may be conceptualised in two different ways. On the one hand, it is an integrationist strategy, which implies that gender issues are addressed within the existing development policy, strategies and priorities. Hence, throughout a project cycle, gender concerns are integrated where applicable. On the other hand, mainstreaming also means agenda setting, which implies transformation of the existing development agenda using a gender perspective. These two concepts are not exclusive and actually work best in combination.

Two other terms which one must understand if the concept of gender mainstreaming is to be grasped, are 'gender perspective' and 'gender-specific policies'.

Gender perspective is a way of (a) analysing and interpreting situations from a viewpoint that takes into consideration the gender constructs in society (for women and men) and (b) searching for solutions to overcome the gaps.

Gender-sensitivity refers to perceptiveness and responsiveness concerning differences in gender roles, responsibilities, challenges and opportunities.

Health care provision should be based on the different needs of women and men. Sometimes this will focus on their biological differences and at other times the emphasis will be on their gender differences. For example, as far as sexual and reproductive health care is concerned, it is recognised that both women and men may need treatment for sexually transmitted infections (STIs) but that only women require services related to safe motherhood and unsafe abortion. Women require facilities for screening and treatment of breast and cervical cancer, while men need facilities for prostate and testicular cancer and less so for breast cancer. Men are more likely to die at a younger age than women due to acute conditions such as coronary artery or cerebro-vascular diseases which are to some extent associated with their gender-based roles. As women live longer, and also because of biological differences, they are more likely to need long-term treatment for chronic conditions such

Health care provision should be based on the different needs of women and men.

A gender-based approach to health care delivery requires an analysis to be made of services provided in order to determine the extent to which they meet the health needs of women and men.

as osteoporosis or arthritis. The different needs of women and men may therefore have a significant impact on the services which are provided for them.

Using Gender Analysis to Define Health Needs

A gender-based approach to health care delivery requires an analysis to be made of services provided in order to determine the extent to which they meet the health needs of women and men. The analysis must take full account of situations such as the following:

- diseases and disabilities from which women suffer because of their sex;

- diseases and disabilities from which both men and women suffer, but which are more prevalent in women;

- diseases and disabilities from which both men and women suffer, but which affect women more severely than men;

- diseases and disabilities from which both men and women suffer, but which have more adverse effects on women during pregnancy;

- diseases and disabilities from which both men and women suffer, but against which women are less able to protect themselves.

Failure to take these factors into account will lead to a situation where the health care system discriminates against women. This will be a violation of international conventions, which prohibit discrimination against women in the provision of health care.

Article 12 of the Convention on the Elimination of All forms of Discrimination Against Women (CEDAW) states:

States Parties shall take all appropriate measures to eliminate discrimination against women in the field of health care in order to ensure, on a basis of equality of men and women, access to health care services, including those related to family planning.

The Beijing Platform for Action states:

Women's right to the enjoyment of the highest standard of health must be secured throughout the whole life cycle in equality with men. The human rights of women include their right to have control over and decide freely and responsibly on matters related to their sexuality, including sexual and reproductive health, free of coercion, discrimination and violence.

The Advocacy for Women's Health Group is a grouping of international health professional associations, reproductive health organisations, women's organisations and women's networks convened by the Commonwealth Medical Association. It has identified some of the diseases and disabilities which fall within the categories mentioned above:

Diseases or disabilities from which women suffer because of their sex

These are mainly conditions affecting the female reproductive system, for example the cervix, uterine body, ovaries and fallopian tubes. Their prevalence, moreover, can provide an important indicator of women's health in the community. They include malignancies, infections and other disorders affecting the female reproductive organs, particularly cervical cancer and pelvic inflammatory disease, as well as eclampsia, ectopic gestation, obstructed labour, uterine inertia, haemorrhage, fistulae and the consequences of unsafe abortion. Disabilities and diseases arising from harmful practices such as female genital mutilation should also be included in this category, as should male violence against women.

Diseases or disabilities from which both men and women suffer, but which are more prevalent in women

These are mainly conditions to which women are more susceptible as a result of their biological differences, compounded by unequal power relationships and unequal access to health resources. They include STIs (which can result in pelvic inflammatory disease, pregnancy-related complications, postpartum morbidity, infections of the newborn, infertility, cancer of the cervix and HIV infection). The consequences to women's health are aggravated in situations where women have relatively poor access to health-care facilities that can deal with such infections. While STIs affect both sexes, women are more susceptible to them for a number of reasons, for example the greater mucosal surface exposed to infection during sexual intercourse and damage to the vaginal mucosa, particularly the immature epithelium in young girls. Women, moreover, are often unaware that they are infected and diagnosis is more difficult as more than half of STIs are asymptomatic (silent) in women. Denial of the right of a woman to insist on safe sexual practices is particularly important in many societies, as HIV infection is far more likely to be transmitted through sexual intercourse if the genital tract is infected by a pre-existing sexually transmitted disease.

In their early and reproductive years, women are also more vulnerable to tuberculosis, which is an indirect cause of many maternal deaths. Urinary schistosomiasis can cause genital lesions that have significant and specific consequences for women, as do various other tropical diseases. Women in all societies suffer cancer of the breast, a condition which is rarely found in men. It may be hormonally or genetically influenced. Women also suffer depressive disorders during the post-natal period. In older life women are more likely than men to suffer from conditions such as arthritis and osteoporosis.

Diseases or disabilities from which men and women suffer, but which have more adverse effects on women during pregnancy

These include diseases and disabilities resulting from poverty and malnutrition, such as pelvic disproportion leading to obstructed labour, uterine inertia and haemorrhage. Diabetes and hypertension are more serious during pregnancy for both mother and foetus. Iron deficiency anaemia, compounded by tropical helminthic infestation and inadequate nutrition, particularly micro-nutrient deficiency, greatly increases the risk to the health of both mother and foetus during pregnancy.

Diseases and disabilities from which both men and women suffer, but against which women are less able to protect themselves

Women are less able to avoid STIs, including HIV/AIDS, as a result both of the difficulty they experience in negotiating safer sex in many societies and of their greater biological susceptibility. The much higher incidence of poverty, malnutrition and illiteracy among women in many societies renders them less able to avoid a wide range of diseases and disabilities, as does their unequal and poorer access to health care facilities.

Gender Inequalities and Women's Health

The unequal power relationship between women and men puts women at a socio-economic disadvantage and this has adverse effects on their health and wellbeing. The following are some of the factors which affect women's health.

Socio-economic factors

The most pervasive consequences of women's socio-economically disadvantaged position are those resulting from poverty: unequal access to health care; lack of information on sexual and reproductive issues and available services; inadequate nutrition; lack of education and gainful employment; and the inability to negotiate safe sex or spacing of pregnancies. Male violence against women, including sexual violence, is also exacerbated by poverty.

There are a number of areas where women, particularly the poorest women, experience gender-related constraints on their access to health services. These include lack of transportation to take them to the services; lack of alternative care for their families while they go for treatment; refusal of the spouse or head of the family to give permission for treatment; lack of sympathetic and culturally appropriate care; and their inability to afford payment for health care for themselves.

Once they have gained access to health care, the quality of care that is provided for women is often inferior to that provided for men and may not reflect their needs. It can also be unnecessarily time-consuming because it is frequently impossible for women to receive treatment themselves at the same time as they take their children for check-ups, immunisations, etc. The services which they receive frequently fail to provide them with an acceptable degree of privacy. They are often not consulted about the treatment they receive and are given little or no information about their health.

Educational factors

The practice of denying female children access to the general education system, widespread in parts of Africa and Asia, is

The most pervasive consequences of women's socio-economically disadvantaged position are those resulting from poverty . . .

. . . the reluctance of many societies to allow girls access to sex education leaves them in ignorance about sexual functions and practices and therefore vulnerable to abuse.

one of the most important determinants of health-related discrimination against women. It results in their being unable to make informed decisions about their own health and that of other members of the family. On an even wider scale, the reluctance of many societies to allow girls access to sex education leaves them in ignorance about sexual functions and practices and therefore vulnerable to abuse. This can have long-term adverse effects on their sexual, reproductive and mental health.

Occupational factors

Women are usually subjected to a 'triple workload', being responsible for all the household tasks and income-generating tasks as well as community tasks. Although male workers die more frequently than female workers from work-related causes, work-related disease among women is increasing in many parts of the world. Jobs that are considered to be 'women's work', such as clerical work, nursing and working in factories and in the free-trade zones, can have adverse physical and psychological effects on women's health. Women also suffer if they take on heavy work which has traditionally been done by men, especially if this is undertaken in combination with work in the home or while the woman is pregnant.

Environmental factors

These include unsafe working conditions in occupations that are mainly carried out by women, for example working on cash crops such as coffee where they are exposed to insecticides, domestic hazards from unsafe cooking stoves which may cause serious burns or respiratory disorders from pollution, and musculo-skeletal disorders arising from the increasing distances which women have to walk to fetch firewood and safe water because environmental pollution and degradation have made nearer sources unusable.

Examples of Gender Discrimination against Women in Health Care Delivery

- Unequal provision of health services for women suffering from diseases or disabilities that affect only women, or are more prevalent in women or affect women differently.

- Failure to take into account the relatively high illiteracy rate of women in many societies when providing health information and services.

- Unequal provision of diagnostic and screening services for women as compared to men for the same groups of diseases and disabilities.

- Unequal provision of resources for research relevant to women, where women and men suffer from the same diseases and disabilities.

- Failure or refusal to provide adolescent girls with access to adequate information about sexual and reproductive health care.

- Laws which deny women access to safe abortion or contraception, or to abortion or sterilisation without spousal consent.

- Failure to ensure that all health services and workers conform to human rights and ethical and gender-sensitive standards in the delivery of women's health services which aim to ensure responsible, voluntary and informed consent.

- Failure to collect sex-disaggregated health data needed to monitor progress in improving the health status of women in the community.

- Failure to take into account differences in the effects of standard doses of prescribed drugs on women, for example body weight, lean body mass and proportion of fat and water.

- Unequal inclusion or absence of women in research

. . . gender roles, reflecting a complex array of forces based on conditioning, custom and peer group pressures, can adversely affect men's health.

Gender Inequalities and Men's Health

It is frequently assumed that gender inequality only affects women's health. On the contrary, it is also necessary to consider what effects gender-based attitudes and behaviour can have on the health of men. Evidence from many countries and societies at different stages of development demonstrates that gender roles, reflecting a complex array of forces based on conditioning, custom and peer group pressures, can adversely affect men's health. The detrimental effects of such gender stereotyping are often further reinforced by the absence of services targeted to meet specific male needs.

In many societies, the sex-based division of labour has forced men to take on tasks which carry risks to health, such as working in mines, using pneumatic drills or working with dangerous chemicals and other hazardous substances. As well as causing long-term ill health, such jobs may carry the risk of accident, thereby contributing to higher occupational mortality and serious injury rates among men.

As men have a higher death rate from acute medical conditions such as cardiovascular or cerebro-vascular episodes, preventive and acute treatment services may be more important for them. It should not be assumed that long-term treatment, which is more appropriate for women, also responds adequately to men's needs. It is also important to increase services for the screening, prevention and treatment of the types of cancer which only men suffer from, for example testicular and prostate cancer.

It is often assumed that existing health services are adequately accessible to men and that men take full advantage of the opportunity to use them. In many cases this is not true. There is a growing awareness that many men fail to make use of the health services altogether or that they only present for treatment when it is too late. The reasons for this type of male behaviour are many and varied. Many men risk their health because of the need to assert their 'masculinity', as they perceive it. Gender-based attitudes encourage a male 'macho' image in which seeking medical help is equated with weakness. Gender stereotyping means that from early childhood many boys and men are conditioned against articulating their problems, anxieties and emotions. Other reasons include the fact that men are often reluctant to take time off work to seek medical attention; they find the location and opening times of health facilities inappropriate and inconvenient; or they find that clinics which are superficially converted from mother and child services and community health services lack the type of structures and male-friendly atmosphere in which they feel comfortable.

3. Gender and Health: Commonwealth Experiences

Introduction

Eight workshops were held in different regions of the Commonwealth:

- **Africa:** Cape Town, South Africa and Entebbe, Uganda
- **Asia:** Colombo, Sri Lanka
- **The Caribbean:** Port of Spain, Trinidad and Tobago, and Frigate Bay, St Kitts and Nevis
- **The South Pacific:** Nadi, Fiji
- Halifax, Canada
- Nicosia, Cyprus

Each workshop was organised by the Health Department of the Commonwealth Secretariat, with the support and participation of its Gender and Youth Affairs Division and in partnership with the Commonwealth Medical Association (CMA).

An important factor in developing a sustainable Gender Management System is the issue of involvement and ownership. A health sector GMS requires close co-operation between many players, both inside and outside the health sector, if it is to achieve its objectives. In addition to the Ministry of Health, several other ministries play a critical role in the provision of facilities and services which impact on the health of the country. If the GMS is intended to set comprehensive norms and practices for the whole health sector, it is important that it also identifies collaborative and supportive roles that can be played by the private sector and NGOs, both of which are key players. In many countries, the private sector is the major provider of health care, at least for those who are insured or who can afford to pay. Some NGOs have a general concern for the health of people, while others may have a particular issue in focus and see their role as maximising efforts to deliver one specialised type of service.

Commonwealth workshops to initiate Gender Management Systems brought together senior policy-makers from Ministries of Health; leading representatives of the health professions; senior officials of Ministries of Women's Affairs, and of Finance or Planning; parliamentary representatives with a health brief and the ability to influence health outcomes; and representatives of national and international NGOs.

Each country delegation to the workshop ideally consisted of 6–10 participants, representing stakeholders at all levels of the health system and reflecting the multisectoral nature of health care. However, for small Commonwealth countries it was not always possible to involve teams of this size and some teams had as few as three or four members. The optimum size for the GMS workshops was judged to be 50–60 participants. The number of participating countries at each workshop varied, ranging from five to eleven.

Workshop Objectives and Methodology

The objectives of the workshops were to:

- examine the concept of the GMS and consider methods of implementing it;

- introduce policy-makers to gender analysis and planning;

- identify key factors associated with gender disparities;

- develop the outline of National Action Plans, which incorporated gender mainstreaming;

- examine opportunities for gender management initiatives to be supported through national, regional and international co-operation.

The proceedings at the workshops were highly participatory in nature and involved a mixture of presentations, discussions and group work, followed by reporting back and debate and reflections on progress. Within each workshop, which lasted for 4–5 days, there were three distinct stages, whose overall aims were:

- to clarify gender concepts;

- to develop an understanding of the concept of the GMS;

- to develop outlines of Plans of Action for a GMS in the health sector.

Clarification of gender concepts

Since the clarification of gender concepts is an essential pre-requisite for developing any plans for gender mainstreaming, a considerable proportion of the workshop time was devoted to this in the first one or two days. The process of enhancing understanding of gender was initiated by short presentations by resource persons, followed by group work in which small groups were asked to discuss and set down definitions of five key concepts:
- gender
- gender sensitivity
- gender analysis
- gender planning
- gender integration/gender mainstreaming.

Each group then reported on their conclusions and consensus developed.

Following this, and having allowed some time for each country team to adjust and refine its material, representatives from each national group were invited to present a Status Report on gender and health in their country against the background of the general constitutional, legal and social situation of women. Presentations included information about national awareness of gender issues, gender policy statements, efforts made to incorporate gender into the public sector and health sector, obstacles and gaps that had been encountered, and positive outcomes and successes. This was followed by discussions in which views and experiences were exchanged about efforts to achieve gender equality in the health sector.

Developing an understanding of the concept of the GMS

Two workshop components contributed to building an understanding of the GMS.

(i) A group exercise was carried out to identify priority health issues for the country/region. Participants applied gender analysis to examine how the gender aspects of this priority health issue would impact on policies, strategies and programme organisation and delivery.

(ii) Formal presentations were made by resource persons to explain the concepts, structures and functions of a GMS in the health sector

Developing outlines of National Plans of Action for establishing the GMS

Participants were urged to view the workshop not as a teacher/learner situation, but rather as one in which knowledge was shared and key concepts clarified as a first step to the development of National Action Plans for the establishment of a GMS. It was emphasised that the purpose was not to impose a ready-made blueprint. Each country would have a different Plan of Action. There was no requirement that the Plan of Action should adopt the GMS approach if it was not deemed suitable. Rather, each country was required to develop the outline of a practical, relevant and tailor-made strategy for mainstreaming gender into the health sector.

Furthermore, participants were reminded that the main outcome of the workshop was not expected to be a complete action plan from each delegation, but rather a framework which would be finalised in their respective countries after discussions with the key stakeholders. It was recognised that final approval and implementation of the Plan of Action was not within the jurisdiction of participants but required government approval, strong political commitment and a broad consensus among stakeholders.

Status of Gender and Health in Commonwealth Regions

Although participants noted that there were variations in health status between countries in the same region, there were more similarities than differences. Variations were wider between regions. The brief summaries of regional health status were not meant to be comprehensive but to give a flavour of the position with regard to gender equality and health as highlighted in the country reports presented at the workshops.

Africa

Two workshops were organised for Africa. The first, held in Cape Town, South Africa, brought together seven countries from the Southern Africa region: Botswana, Lesotho, Mozambique, Namibia, South Africa, Swaziland and Zimbabwe. The level of national gender awareness appeared to be generally high, particularly in urban areas. All the countries had ratified the Convention on the Elimination of All Forms of Discrimination Against Women and most of them had set up machinery to address gender issues. However, in none of them was gender equality treated as a special issue in the health sector.

The second workshop for Africa was held in Entebbe, Uganda. Nine countries were represented: Cameroon, The Gambia, Ghana, Kenya, Malawi, Sierra Leone, Tanzania, Uganda and Zambia. Participants noted that Africa had made some progress towards addressing women's issues. However, in spite of major efforts, gender imbalances continued to exist. All the countries were signatories to CEDAW. Efforts were being made to increase national gender awareness and all countries had taken action to set up some machinery to address gender issues. Indeed, some countries were already piloting national Gender Management Systems. Most participants recognised the need for gender mainstreaming in the health sector and acknowledged that so far health programmes had tended to benefit women and children.

Asia

Participants from five Asian countries attended the workshop in Colombo, Sri Lanka: Bangladesh, India, Malaysia, Pakistan and Sri Lanka. Participants observed that although women generally tended to occupy a subordinate position in society, efforts were being made to promote gender equality through policies, media publicity, collection of sex-disaggregated data, etc. All the countries had signed CEDAW and had established National Women's Machineries to promote women's issues and gender equality. However, a gap still existed between policy and societal attitudes.

Health programmes had tended to focus on maternal and child health. One country had moved on to establish Family Health Programmes. In some countries, women were not employed in key ministries because of a lack of education and training or because of a failure to appreciate the potential contribution that they could make. Women were traditionally employed in the health sector but were conspicuously absent from key and senior positions. This was partly due to pressures of domestic duties, and partly to institutions which were set up to suit male working patterns and therefore lacked the flexibility which women required.

The Caribbean

The first workshop was held in Port of Spain, Trinidad and Tobago. Eight Caribbean countries participated: Barbados, Belize, Guyana, Jamaica, St Lucia, St Kitts and Nevis, St Vincent and the Grenadines, and Trinidad and Tobago.

The overall impression was that considerable progress had been made in advancing gender issues in government, society and the health sector. This was evident in new legislation, the setting up of women's bureaux, the introduction of Gender Focal Points in ministries and the establishment of government machinery such as National Action Plans and Steering Committees to mainstream gender into policies and programmes. Initiatives had been introduced to sensitise people to gender equality and to target key gender issues. The media had been used as a tool in these efforts. Attention had been focused on gender-related health problems such as breast or cervical cancer.

The second Caribbean workshop took place in St Kitts and Nevis. Eleven countries were represented: Anguilla, Antigua and Barbuda, British Virgin Islands, Cayman Islands, Dominica, Grenada, Monserrat, St Kitts and Nevis, St Vincent and the Grenadines, Turks and Caicos, and Canada.

It was again noted that the Caribbean region had made significant progress in addressing women's issues, although this was not to be interpreted as having resolved gender imbalances, which continued to exist. It was encouraging to note the high level of national awareness on gender issues. All countries were signatories to CEDAW and had taken steps to set up some machinery for addressing gender issues. St Kitts and Nevis was in the process of piloting a national GMS and this provided some practical insights into the advantages and disadvantages of the system. The need for a system to mainstream gender into the health sector was clear to most participants. They agreed that nearly all health programmes tended to benefit women and children, while omitting any specific focus on men's health.

The South Pacific

The GMS workshop in the Pacific region was held in Fiji, 19-23 October 1998. For many Pacific Island States, gender and gender issues were new and the level of awareness among the general public was low.

In the government sector some employees had been given gender sensitisation training. However, gender was not being given higher priority and greater political will was needed to ensure a higher level of participation of women in decision-making. One of the main obstacles was societal/cultural; norms in which roles and responsibilities of males and females are determined by society and perpetuated within the social structure and handed down traditionally "without question".

Despite this some positive actions were being taken such as the setting up of a gender support facility in Tonga and the integration of gender issues into the project cycles guidelines.

A number of agencies had been assisting the efforts to prioritise gender in the Pacific region. The Pacific Women's Resource Bureau of the Secretariat Pacific Community, UNDP and UNIFEM had been involved in activities such as gender audit, development of gender policies and strategies and mainstreaming efforts.

Countries with multi-jurisdictional governance

A workshop held in Halifax, Nova Scotia, Canada was attended by four countries: Canada, India, Nigeria and South

Africa. Participants came from countries with widely differing population sizes and stages of development but they had some common features, including the fact that they were all multi-jurisdictional states.

South Africa reported that the new South Africa had inherited a public service characterised by discriminatory employment polices and practices based on race, gender and disability. One of the government's foremost challenges was to transform the public service into an efficient and effective instrument for delivering an equitable service to all citizens, using a gender-sensitive and non-discriminatory approach. The National Gender Machinery had been set up to improve the position of South African women. The National Department of Health had adopted a strategy to change attitudes and assumptions which impede the achievement of gender equality in the health sector.

Nigeria reported that its Constitution guarantees rights on the basis of equality between women and men, and also provides instruments for enforcement. However, this was at variance with various cultural practices in the country where a system based on patriarchy accorded superiority to men. Women were therefore significantly disadvantaged. There was little awareness of the importance of gender issues among the general public and even health workers were not always very gender-sensitive, a factor which had contributed to increasing maternal and child mortality rates.

India reported that its population was growing at an extremely fast rate and was expected to cross the one billion mark in 2000. There had been a significant change in the female/male ratio in the population; this was the result of son-preference and the historical neglect of health care for women. The higher death rates for women in all age groups were a phenomenon unique to India. There was a need for much better health care for girl-children, adolescent girls and women in the reproductive age group. India's Constitution incorporated fundamental rights without discrimination, including gender discrimination. Social problems created by the dowry system were still evident but an Anti-Dowry Act had been passed, though the onus of proof rested with the defendant. The Department of Women and Children managed a major nutritional programme and promoted affirmative schemes for girl-children, education for women and women's position in politics. The Maternal and Child Health Programme was decentralised, client-driven and gender-sensitive.

Canada reported that the country did not have national machinery. Its presentation was therefore divided into sections on the Federal approach to health, a provincial approach, a perspective on aboriginal health and the relationship between the Federal government and the NGO community. Gender balance remained one of the biggest challenges because gender was still seen as a women's issue. Canada had a government-wide Federal Plan for gender equality which committed all Federal departments and agencies to ensure that all new legislation and policies were analysed for their differential impact on women and men, where appropriate. Health Canada, which operated at federal level, had identified 12 inter-related determinants of health. Gender was seen as a determinant in its own right as well as one that cut across and influenced all other determinants.

The **Cyprus** workshop identified a number of positive measures which had been taken to mainstream gender both at the national level and in the health sectors of participating countries, all of which were small states. All the countries had a strong focus on women's issues and saw CEDAW as one of the most important international legal instruments under which women's rights have been recognised as human rights. Action taken to mainstream gender had been guided by CEDAW, the Beijing Plan of Action and the Commonwealth Plan of Action on Gender and Development. All the countries had established National Women's Machineries although some were more active than others.

Participants indicated that the level of awareness of gender had increased considerably in recent years. Much more needed to be done, however, to ensure equity of access to health care and the development of more appropriate health services for both women and men.

A number of structures have been established in Cyprus to support the new focus on gender. For example, a Gender Equality Council, headed by the President, replaced the National Women's Council in 2000.

The main challenges facing the countries were the lack of technical expertise and funds to advance the gender mainstreaming process, and a discrepancy between rhetoric and action at high political and administrative levels in some of the countries.

Positive initiatives towards gender mainstreaming in health

Several countries referred to positive initiatives which had been taken to support gender mainstreaming in health:

- The enactment of key legislation on gender equality and women's human rights;

- Statements by leading politicians in support of gender equality;

- The establishment of National Women's Machineries, Women's Affairs Departments, Women's Bureaux and Gender Focal Points;

- The establishment of various kinds of government machinery to mainstream gender, for example National Gender Action Councils and Gender Steering Committees;

- Use of the media, radio, television, newspapers, etc. to increase public awareness of gender issues;

- Emphasis on health initiatives which address gender-related problems, for example breast, cervical and prostate cancer screening;

- Targeting health programmes at vulnerable groups which might be encountering gender-related health problems, for example by setting up refugee and crisis centres for victims of violence, sexual abuse and rape;

- Reaching out to men by using male counsellors.

Critical Issues and Challenges

Critical issues

At each of the workshops, participants and resource persons worked together to identify some of the critical gender issues and challenges facing countries in the provision of health services. Some of the issues were emphasised by only a few countries, while others were relevant for nearly every country. Views which were expressed are summarised below.

. . . differences in the way in which society treats girls and boys can lead to different lifestyles in adulthood which then impact on their life expectancies.

Attitudes to gender issues

It was agreed that negative attitudes to gender issues should be changed. Gender issues were rooted in social constructs rather than in biological fact, so gender-based attitudes were the product of learned behaviour, and could and should be changed through appropriate education, sensitisation and training. The challenge of bringing about the necessary changes could be taken up by introducing gender mainstreaming into the health sector.

Examples of gender inequality in the health sector

Instances of gender inequality in health, which have hitherto been accepted with complacency, should be subjected to gender analysis. This could lead to the identification of some of the underlying causes of the inequalities and to prompt action to remedy the situation. For example, data for one region revealed that the average life expectancies of populations had varied in the past by about 10 years. This was obviously a health issue. However, a new dimension was added when the data were disaggregated by sex. This showed that in every country women had longer life expectancies than men by a margin of 2–7 years.

If a biology-based approach is taken, one is likely to simply accept the status quo on the basis that this happens in the majority of countries in the world and that therefore women are probably biologically designed to live longer than men. In that case there would be no problem to be investigated and solved. However, if a gender-based approach is taken, then further gender analysis is justified. This might well open up other possible explanations which could then be subjected to further research. Tracing the problem back to birth, one might observe that in many countries there is a tendency for son-preference, so baby boys get more food and attention than girls. This information becomes significant when it is viewed in the context of evidence that nutritional patterns in early childhood may have a profound effect on health problems in adult life. The possibility then arises that overfeeding and over-indulgence of boys may establish a preference for larger helpings and fatty foods being given to boys and men, thus laying the foundation of increased risk of cardiovascular and skeleto-motor diseases.

Attitudes to risk-taking present another example of how gender-based differences in expectations of girls and boys can affect their health differently in adult life. In many cultures, boys are generally encouraged to be active, adventurous and daring, while girls are expected to be relatively cautious, careful and responsible. This pattern, which is established in childhood, is carried into adulthood. Men, more than women, are expected to engage in dangerous work, which exposes them to physical injury. They then require health care as a result of the consequences of their exposure to such risks, some of which may be life-threatening or fatal.

This illustrates how differences in the way in which society treats girls and boys can lead to different lifestyles in adulthood which then impact on their life expectancies. This should lead planners to consider how gender-sensitive planning and gender mainstreaming could affect life expectancies. Planners and researchers would need to examine the biological, as well as the socially-constructed, aspects of the lives of women and men in order to identify factors which are shortening their life expectancies. The issue would not be a competition to see whether it was women or men who would live longer but to eliminate any factors which reduce the life expectancies of both women and men. The data collected would then be used to make gender-sensitive interventions to increase life expectancies for everyone. These interventions might be different for women and men because of their different needs, lifestyles and constraints. In this way, gender-based research and planning can benefit both women and men.

There are many other instances where gender analysis can be useful for understanding health issues which relate to both women and men. Whenever we look at sex-disaggregated data, whether it is on incidences of disease, reasons for death, causes of disability, patterns of use of health services at primary, secondary and tertiary levels, expenditure on health systems, facilities and services, or employment of women and men at different levels and in various branches of the health sector, we need to consider what the data actually mean in our quest for gender equality. Prior assumptions should be reviewed and in each case meticulous gender analysis should be applied. Only then can the most appropriate intervention for any particular population be determined.

. . . if there is a narrow and exclusive focus on women as childbearers, it perpetuates the stereotyping of women as mothers.

Many actions which have a major impact on health are the responsibility of sectors outside the health sector.

Differences in ranges of health programmes

Although many countries have addressed health programmes across a wide spectrum of issues, some have operated at another extreme where health care is focused almost exclusively on women, and more so on women's reproductive role. Dr Mahnoud Fathalla, former Director of the World Health Organisation's Special Programme of Research Training in Human Reproductive gave a warning against the narrow position in the following statements:

A women is not a womb: a woman has a womb.

Pregnancy is not a disease: it is a special event in a women's life, but one to which serious risks are attached.

Undoubtedly, maternal and child health programmes are vital and respond to the needs of women and children during pregnancy, childbirth, infancy and childhood. However, if there is a narrow and exclusive focus on women as childbearers, it perpetuates the stereotyping of women as mothers. This can limit women's freedom of choice as individuals and also deprive them of services which they need at other stages of their lives, for example puberty, adolescence, menopause and old age. Furthermore, this exclusive focus excludes men from health services that they need.

Challenges

Participants referred to many gaps and challenges facing the health sector as it has tried to mainstream gender into its policies and programmes. Reference has already been made to some of the key problems identified by countries:

- Lack of political commitment;

- Lack of sensitisation to gender issues among the public;

- Lack of training for decision-makers, implementers and other officials;

- Inefficient and limited information and data collection systems;

- Marginalisation of men, for example men were not sufficiently involved in issues to do with reproductive responsibility or child rearing and inadequate attention was paid to health issues affecting men.

Other examples of gaps and challenges identified by countries are given below.

Underlying gender and health issues are intersectoral

Many of the underlying issues relating to gender and health are intersectoral in nature. Many actions which have a major impact on health are the responsibility of sectors outside the health sector. For example, within government in sectors such as finance, education, transport, water and sanitation, employment and social welfare, decisions are taken which have a major and often differential impact on the health of women and men. Societal, cultural and traditional attitudes may also have a significant differential impact on health by encouraging or discouraging certain types of behaviour, or by denying or underplaying the importance of certain issues. Inter-ministerial co-ordinating committees and similar mechanisms can be used to achieve intersectoral co-ordination. However, it is usually difficult to achieve this satisfactorily, especially because there are budgetary implications when work is shared between ministries.

Fragmented health services

Health services are often fragmented. This leads to gaps in provision and coverage. This can happen when, for instance, a decision is taken to alter an existing service or to introduce a new service but this is done in a piecemeal manner or without reference to other aspects of the health care system. The result has often been that even if the new service meets its own targets, some other part of the system has deteriorated as a result of shifts in priorities and resource allocation. This strengthens the case for looking at the health sector as a whole and adopting a more comprehensive and integrated approach to planning. If the planning is based on a proper assessment of needs and an equitable distribution of resources, then the dangers resulting from fragmentation are likely to be reduced.

Lack of resources

Lack of resources remains one of the major obstacles to progress.

Lack of resources remains one of the major obstacles to progress. The reality is that in every country all aspects of the health sector are under-resourced.

The reality is that in every country all aspects of the health sector are under-resourced. The critical issue then becomes how priorities are to be set so that work can continue in spite of constraints imposed by the lack of resources. In such a situation, any attempt to treat women's health or gender mainstreaming as a separate issue requiring its own budget will invariably lead to heated arguments about the displacement of other competing needs. It could be contended that treating women's issues or gender issues as separate issues from other major health issues, such as communicable and non-communicable diseases or deciding whether hospitals can be kept open, can jeopardise attention to gender and health issues. To avoid this controversy over paucity of resources, it should be emphasised that gender mainstreaming seeks to find the most efficient ways of using existing resources by focusing on the needs of both women and men. The position then becomes not so much one of focusing on a disadvantaged group as of implementing the most equitable and efficient use of resources so as to provide the best level of healthcare for women and men. This would put into effect the statement that:

Health is a fundamental right and it must be accessible to all and universal in its application.

Inadequate monitoring and evaluation systems
Monitoring and evaluation systems are often weak and it is not always clear what monitoring and evaluation mechanisms are appropriate. Consequently, it is difficult to assess the impact of gender mainstreaming initiatives or to determine the extent to which the objective of equality of outcomes for both women and men is being achieved. It is easier to carry out monitoring and evaluation if this is limited to statistical data. This could involve statistics on numbers of health workers by sex, numbers of patients treated by sex, etc. However, this would not address underlying differences and inequalities, and would therefore be insufficient. Monitoring and evaluation therefore remains a serious challenge in attempts to measure the impact of gender mainstreaming in the health sector.

Gap between policy and implementation
There is often a gap between policy and implementation in the sense that strong policy statements are made and supporting

legislation is put in place, but this still does not guarantee that effective action will be taken.

Gap between awareness and attitudes

There is often a gap between awareness and attitudes. It is often observed that even where there is a high level of gender awareness, this is not followed by the desired change in attitudes or behaviour. It has proved much easier for the health system to put services which are designed to be gender-sensitive in place, than to bring about a change in attitudes. This is disturbing because real and sustained change cannot be achieved in the health sector unless all stakeholders, providers as well as users, adopt gender-sensitive attitudes.

Inadequate training in gender analysis and planning

Relatively few people in the health sector have received training in gender analysis and planning, both of which are tools required for pursuing a gender and development approach. Yet it is clear that the design and implementation of health policies and programmes require an understanding of gender issues by all key players, and not just by a few experts. This is a worldwide problem as highlighted at the Hague International Forum held in 1999 to review progress on the International Conference on Population and Development (ICPD) Programme of Action. The draft report on Incorporation of a Gender Perspective concluded:

The adoption of this approach has been hampered by the absence of a proper understanding of how to interpret concepts related to gender issues in different social and cultural contexts.

The problem is aggravated by the fact that there are very few good training materials, and even fewer courses, on gender issues, that are appropriate for use with the broad range of workers in the health sector. Yet these are the people responsible for the implementation of a new gender-aware health care service. The international community is therefore faced with a major problem in its efforts to support countries in the process of mainstreaming gender into their health sectors.

Some international organisations, such as the United Nations Population Fund (UNFPA), Pan American Health Organisation (PAHO) and the Commonwealth Secretariat, as

Male involvement in the process of gender mainstreaming in the health sector is essential.

well as some bilateral agencies in North America and Europe, have developed training materials on gender, primarily or partly for use by their own staff and consultants. These materials can be used with appropriate adaptations by health personnel. The fact remains that materials are very limited. The Commonwealth Secretariat has tried to fill this gap by publishing a *Gender and Health Curriculum Guide* for teaching programmes in about 15 topics relating to gender and health. It is hoped that this will be used in teaching/training institutions around the world. Avenues are also being sought for establishing teaching programmes based on the *Curriculum Guide*. There will be an emphasis on the use of distance education methodologies so that the courses are accessible to health workers wherever they are located.

Inadequate male involvement

Male involvement in the process of gender mainstreaming in the health sector is essential. The focus is often on increasing women's role in decision-making. Yet without a change in male attitudes, so that men become supportive of gender mainstreaming, the entire process will be in jeopardy.

The Gender Perspective on Priority Setting

Participants at the various workshops met in groups to identify priority issues in the health sector. Each group then worked on one of these priority issues identifying appropriate action with regard to health policies, programmes, service delivery strategy, recruitment and training of health personnel and their terms and conditions of employment, health information systems and financial resources. An overriding consideration in the discussion on each issue was to decide on the gender issues involved and to determine what interventions would lead to equality between women and men.

In the case of the Caribbean workshops, because Caribbean Ministers of Health had a meeting just before the workshop and had already identified priority issues for the region, these were used by participants as the basis for discussion. Priority issues identified by some of the regions were as follows.

Workshop held in South Africa

Reproductive health; adolescent health; ageing; nutrition;

HIV/AIDS; other communicable diseases, including tuber-culosis and malaria.

Workshop held in Sri Lanka

Reproductive health; nutrition; violence against women; sub-stance abuse; HIV/AIDS.

Workshops held in the Caribbean

Environmental health; solid and liquid waste management; chronic non-communicable diseases; mental health; family health; prevention and control of communicable diseases, including HIV/AIDS; food and nutrition.

Workshop held in Cyprus

HIV/AIDS and other STDs; sexual health; non-communicable diseases; mental health; substance abuse; violence; osteo-porosis; accidents.

Workshop held in Uganda

Malaria; HIV/AIDS and STIs; diarrhoeal diseases; respiratory tract infections; tuberculosis; meningitis; malnutrition; mater-nal and perinatal mortality and morbidity; anaemia; trauma and gender-based violence, including female genital mutila-tion; hypertension; diabetes; cancer; onchocerciasis and tropi-cal diseases; leprosy; depression and anxiety disorders.

Subjecting health issues to gender analysis proved to be a use-ful exercise for participants. It underlined the need for coun-tries to carry out more intensive and focused analyses, set up better information systems using sex-disaggregated data, and to formulate relevant policies and implement well-managed pro-grammes and processes to improve gender equality in the health sector.

4. Establishing the Gender Management System in the Health Sector

Introduction

The Commonwealth Secretariat's *Gender Management System Handbook* defines the GMS as follows:

A Gender Management System (GMS) is a network of structures, mechanisms and processes put in place within an existing organisational framework, to guide, plan, monitor and evaluate the process of mainstreaming gender into all areas of the organisation's work, in order to achieve greater gender equality and equity within the context of sustainable development. A GMS may be established at any level of government, or in institutions such as universities, intergovernmental or non-governmental organisations, private sector organisations or trade unions.

The description of the process of establishing a GMS in the health sector given in this publication will be guided by the generic definition as given above. Reference may be made to the *Gender Management System Handbook* for a more detailed description of the generic GMS.

A GMS in health may be implemented at different levels, national, provincial, regional or local, or for an individual institution or NGO whose work focuses on health issues.

Integrating gender into the health sector through a GMS will involve other sectors of government as the health sector does not function in isolation. Its work is inter-related with that of other sectors. The issue of nutrition and health, for example, can overlap with the interests and priorities of Ministries of Agriculture, Trade, Education, Transportation, Information, Labour and Social Services.

When a GMS is to be introduced, it is important to take stock of national and local realities and needs. Country status reports will be useful in providing the context within which the GMS will operate. These could include reports which have been prepared by the government as part of its reporting obligations to CEDAW; reports prepared for the UN Commission on the Status of Women as part of the process of monitoring implementation of the Beijing Platform for Action; reports prepared by NGOs; National Development Plans; country status reports prepared by UN agencies such as the UNDP and UNICEF; and other regional, national and local reports on the status of women in general or on women's health.

Vision, Mission and Goals

Vision

The vision towards which the government is working is 'a health sector in which women and men have equal rights and opportunities and both are respected and valued as equal and able partners at all levels of the health system'. Within this framework 'women and men will work in collaboration and partnership, utilising their full potential to ensure that the specific health needs of all are adequately met and all health policies, programmes and procedures are gender-sensitive'.

Mission

The mission of a GMS in the health sector is to achieve gender equality and equity through strategic action such as securing political will, forging a partnership among stakeholders, building capacity and promoting good practices in gender mainstreaming.

Goal

The goal of a GMS in the health sector is to ensure the integration of gender into all government policies, programmes and activities which impact on health.

Objectives

The objectives of a GMS in the health sector are to:

- Build capacity in the Ministry of Health to draw up gender-aware policies and plans for the development of all levels of the health sector. Such policies will impact on recruitment, continuing education and training, terms and conditions of service, and health care programmes;

- Build capacity in all relevant ministries and agencies to ensure that any policies and programmes which are initiated and which affect the health of the population take gender concerns fully into account;

- Facilitate partnership between all organisations which influence health outcomes – government ministries and departments, intergovernmental organisations, the private sector and NGOs;

- Support gender equality and equity through education and the promotion of the concepts among providers and users of health services;

- Provide an enabling environment for effective implementation, monitoring and evaluation of gender mainstreaming in health policies and programmes in both the public and private sectors.

The GMS as a Management Tool

Gender mainstreaming is based on the development assumptions that gender equality/equity is a variable which is central to national development; a human rights issue that stands for fairness and social justice for women and men in society; a core element of good governance through people-oriented, participatory management; and an enabling factor in efforts to alleviate poverty and all its social consequences.

Within the context of these development assumptions, gender mainstreaming is an integrative process, which is:

- Seeking to transform existing unequal gender relations into relations of equality and equity by addressing the root causes of gender gaps and disparities in all sectors; ascertaining whether it is women or men who are at a disadvantage in a particular situation; addressing practical and strategic needs from the different perspectives of women and men; empowering both women and men; and improving social relationships between the two genders;

- Context-specific, taking into account the socio-economic, political, institutional and cultural framework of the society;

- Systems-wide, thus regarding the achievement of gender

equality not as the exclusive concern of women but as the shared responsibility of the entire society, and specifically of the public sector in collaboration with non-state agencies;

- Needs-based and information driven, based on quantitative and qualitative gender-aware research and analysis;

- Oriented to inputs/outputs/outcomes, i.e. impact assessment;

- Resource-sensitive and cost-effective.

The GMS employs a methodology, which focuses on the four Ms: Mainstreaming, Multitracking, Management and Measurement.

- **Mainstreaming:** the entire state sector, in collaboration with non-state stakeholders, is responsible and accountable for achieving specified gender equality/equity goals and objectives, with the National Women's Machinery playing a catalytic role.

- **Multitracking:** there is a need to track the gaps and inequalities between women and men in all sectors through sex-disaggregated data and qualitative gender analysis, and address the differential needs and interests of women and men. This must be done within a framework of internationally agreed goals and objectives that guide the thrust toward gender equality/equity.

- **Management:** emphasises both the technical tasks of mainstreaming gender into policy formulation, development planning and service delivery, and the administrative procedures and change management processes required for so doing.

- **Measurement:** ensures not just equality of inputs in terms of policy initiatives and service delivery but, critically, equality of outcomes and impacts on the quality of life of both women and men. The use of sector-based gender-sensitive indicators constitutes a vital tool to be used for this purpose.

The GMS thus seeks to facilitate the process of institutional change from 'gender-blind' and 'gender-neutral' to 'gender-aware' and 'gender-specific' policies, plans and programmes.

Gender-neutral policies, plans and programmes rely on accurate information about the existing gender-based division of resources and responsibilities in order to ensure that the policy and programmes objectives (whether related to production or welfare) are met in the most efficient way. Gender-neutral policies, plans and programmes presume that women and men play complementary roles within the social division of labour. Such policies, plans and programmes address practical, as opposed to strategic, gender needs of women and men; allocate resources to women and men for the efficient and effective execution of their roles/responsibilities; leave the existing division of resources and responsibilities intact; and ignore the power differentials that exist between women and men in decision-making at all levels.

Gender-aware or **gender-sensitive** or **gender-transformative** policies, plans and programmes are those which seek to transform existing gender relations to relations of equality and equity by redistributing more evenly the division of resources, responsibilities and power between women and men. Gender-aware policies, plans and programmes have the following advantages: they are empowering to both women and men; they lead to improved social relationships between women and men; they address the root causes of gender gaps and disparities, and forms of discrimination in all sectors of development; and they address both practical and strategic gender needs from the perspectives of women and men in a complementary manner.

Gender-specific policies, plans and programmes usually address specific gender gaps or forms of discrimination from the standpoint of women's or men's specific gender needs or interests. Gender-specific policies, plans and programmes are the quickest method of reducing practical and strategic gender gaps and forms of discrimination between women and men in any sector. However, without some transformative potential built into them, gender-specific policies, plans and programmes are likely to leave the existing division of resources and responsibilities intact, and to fail to sensitise women about existing gender gaps and discrimination in the sector being addressed. This means that while, laudably, practical gender needs are being addressed and even met, the strategic issues that would transform the relationship between women and men in the given sector are left untouched.

Figure 1. The Gender Management System

Enabling Environment

- Political will
- Adequate human and financial resources
- Legislative and administrative framework
- Active involvement of civil society

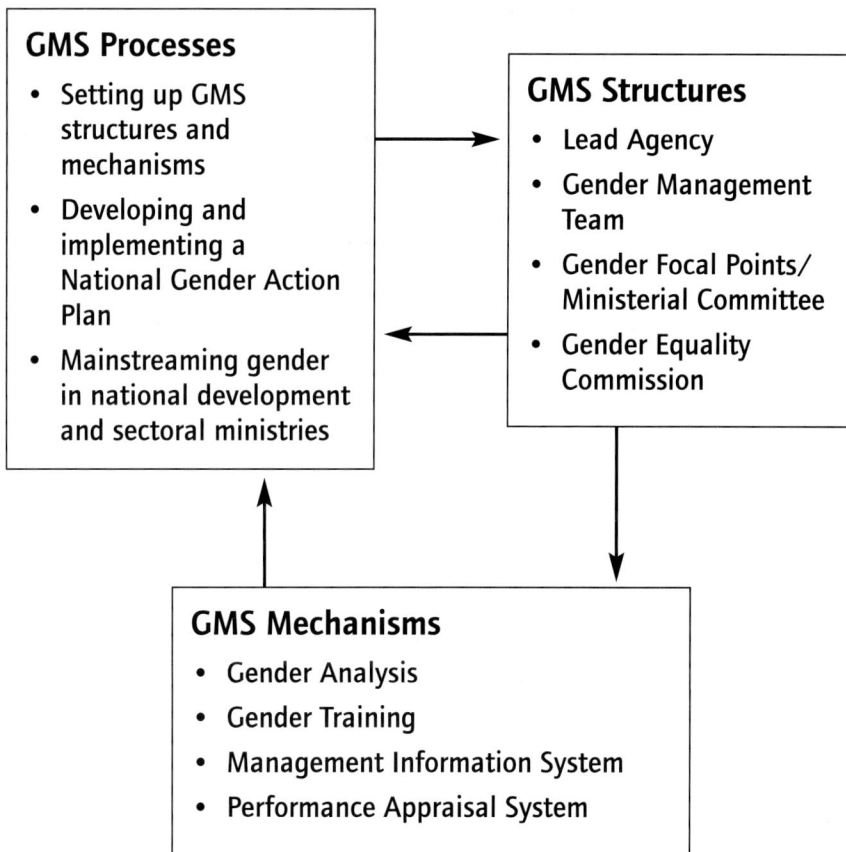

GMS Processes

- Setting up GMS structures and mechanisms
- Developing and implementing a National Gender Action Plan
- Mainstreaming gender in national development and sectoral ministries

GMS Structures

- Lead Agency
- Gender Management Team
- Gender Focal Points/ Ministerial Committee
- Gender Equality Commission

GMS Mechanisms

- Gender Analysis
- Gender Training
- Management Information System
- Performance Appraisal System

Source: *Gender Mainstreaming in Science and Technology*, Commonwealth Secretariat, 2001.

A GMS in the health sector cannot be effective . . . if there is not an enabling environment.

The Structures, Mechanisms and Processes of the GMS

The enabling environment for the GMS

Reference has already been made to the importance of creating an enabling environment for the GMS in any sector. A GMS in the health sector cannot be effective, and indeed may not take off, if there is not an enabling environment. Political commitment to the whole process of mainstreaming gender in the health sector is vital. This is important in many countries where the traditional approach, which has public appeal, is to deliver health care which targets women and children in the form of reproductive health care, maternal and child care, etc. Another approach which is popular is to focus on a general programme for improving hospital services. Gender mainstreaming is a new approach, which initially might not have the same popularity as the former WID approach and may not, therefore, immediately appeal to politicians.

One of the first tasks facing the Ministry of Health is to secure political and public endorsement of the GMS as a mechanism for making health delivery more efficient, equitable and responsive to the different needs of women and men. The Ministry must work towards winning acceptance of the fact that with the GMS approach women and men become equal contributors to, and beneficiaries of, the health service.

Supportive legislative and administrative frameworks also contribute to the enabling environment. It is easier for a Ministry of Health to justify the adoption of the gender mainstreaming approach used in the GMS if a country is signatory to the international conventions which advocate gender equality and equity, for example CEDAW, the Beijing Platform for Action and ICPD. It is also supportive to have a national constitution and national legislation which prohibit discrimination on the grounds of sex, promote equity and equality between women and men, and protect women's human rights as an integral part of human rights.

If these enabling factors are present, they will facilitate the setting up of a GMS in the health sector. The Ministry will then find it easier to get support for providing gender-sensitive health care. For instance, there could be a focus on women who have been victims of domestic violence and sexual abuse. In the context of the GMS model, the Ministry of Health will not only devote its own resources to treating the women, but will have a better framework for liaising with other relevant services, such as the police and social services, which are also involved in responding to the needs of women who have suffered domestic violence.

GMS structures

Stakeholders

A GMS is a co-operative initiative involving stakeholders or partners strategically placed to bring about gender equity and equality. Stakeholders in a GMS in the health sector will include all ministries, but especially the ministries of health, finance and planning, women's/gender affairs, social services, education, transportation, information, employment, agriculture, environment and justice. Other stakeholders include NGOs, particularly women's organisations, development agencies, the media, trade unions, professional associations, university and research institutions, donor agencies, the private sector and the beneficiaries themselves.

Primary stakeholders are those most affected, either positively or negatively, by the system. In the health sector, recipients and providers of health care may also be considered as primary stakeholders. Gender discrimination is not limited to recipients or providers who are in the formal structure of the health sector. It may also affect the large number of people, mainly women, who work as carers at home and in institutions.

Lead agency

The Ministry of Health will normally be the lead agency in the implementation of a GMS in the health sector. However, the cross-sectoral nature of a GMS and the requirements for collaboration with other ministries and civil society make close participation by a range of other stakeholders essential. While the precise roles and responsibilities of each partner will be unique to each country (or even to each province, in the case of multi-jurisdictional states) and will need to be defined precisely in the course of negotiating and developing each jurisdiction's own action plan, a number of general points and principles can be set out for guidance.

As lead agency, the Ministry of Health will take overall responsibility for developing and implementing the GMS in the health sector. A division or unit within the ministry may be given responsibility for co-ordinating implementation of the Plan of Action.

The functions of the lead agency are described in the GMS *Handbook* as follows:

The Lead Agency initiates and strengthens the institutional arrangements of the GMS and is responsible for the overall co-ordination and monitoring of the GMS. It advocates for change and works to impact upon policy decision. It plays a strategic and catalytic role, introducing critical gender concerns into the policies, plans and programmes of the core and sectoral government agencies, ensuring that key targets and indicators on the status of women are agreed upon and met, managing the flow of information on gender issues and communicating policy changes and results.

Gender Management Team
A Gender Management Team should be set up composed of the Permanent Secretary of the Ministry of Health (as the representative from the lead agency) and permanent secretaries from key ministries and representatives of civil society. The responsibilities of the Gender Management Team were outlined in the GMS *Handbook* as follows:

The Gender Management Team's responsibility includes developing the GMS concept ... providing the GMS with broad operational policies, indicators of effectiveness and timeframes for implementation. The Team should seek to expand the scope of gender mainstreaming.

Gender Focal Points
The profile of Gender Focal Points as described in the GMS *Handbook* is as follows:

Gender Focal Points are designated senior members of staff within each ministry/department /division who are either directly involved in, or able to influence, their sector's planning process.

Some of the functions of Gender Focal Points are:

- Supporting and encouraging colleagues so that gender-sensitive policies and programmes are developed within their own ministry/department /division;

- Acting as in-house advocates and providing expert advice to colleagues on gender mainstreaming in all their work in the context of the GMS Action Plan;

- Supporting and promoting the application of gender analysis to all policies and programmes in their ministry/department and division;

- Collecting and disseminating information and best practices on gender mainstreaming;

- Supporting the development and use of an efficient information system on gender mainstreaming;

- Supporting the monitoring and evaluation processes set up to assess implementation of the GMS.

Mechanisms of the GMS

Gender analysis

The collection and analysis of sex-disaggregated data is a prerequisite for efficient planning and implementation of a GMS in health. Without such data, it is impossible for planners to ensure that they know what the different needs of women and men are so that appropriate health care can be provided for them.

Gender training

Training in gender mainstreaming is necessary for all staff members at all levels in the Ministry of Health. It will also be required for all other officials in other ministries and collaborating institutions and organisations whose work impacts on the establishment of a GMS in health. Gender-awareness training should also be provided for the general public because they are the beneficiaries of health care and are also carers in the community.

Health management information system

Participants at the Commonwealth workshops identified this as a gap in the provision of a comprehensive service. An efficient gender management information system would assemble and disseminate information on the GMS as well as on other gender mainstreaming, gender equality and gender equity issues.

Performance appraisal system

A gender-sensitive performance appraisal system should be set up in the Ministry of Health to measure changes in individual and departmental standards of achievement of the goals of the GMS, including the extent to which individual staff members have acquired gender awareness and applied such awareness in their work.

GMS processes

The following are three inter-related processes in the establishment of a GMS in health:

- Establishing GMS structures and mechanisms (as outlined above);

- Developing and implementing a Gender Action Plan for integrating gender into health and developing appropriate monitoring and evaluation mechanisms;

- Mainstreaming gender into national development plans and into the sectoral plans, policies and programmes of other relevant or collaborating ministries and stakeholders.

Factors which Hinder the Establishment of a GMS in Health

Lack of gender-sensitive indicators

Many countries, especially developing countries, lack basic information on the different ways in which women and men are affected by ill health and how differences in age affect the health of both women and men. National health statistics often fail to distinguish between women and men in recording data. Yet efficient gender-sensitive planning is impossible without such basic information. There is, therefore, an urgent need for those countries which do not provide data by both age and sex to start doing so.

The problem created by the lack of such data can be seen, for example, when it is known that older women or young girls are at risk from particular health problems which the health sector wants to address by monitoring their nutritional status and their access to health care. If there is no database from which the relevant information on these target groups can be accessed, health workers cannot easily monitor them or provide comprehensive and timely health care from which all would benefit. Similarly, if there are no sex-disaggregated data on special groups of disadvantaged women such as migrants, refugees, single heads of households, or people suffering from chronic diseases or long-term disability, health workers cannot easily set up programmes which respond to these women's special health needs.*

In some developing countries, there is no systematic registration of live births or stillbirths. Indeed, in some rural areas there may not be any system of registration. This means that there is no reliable database on the country's age profile or on infant mortality rates; this makes planning of better maternal and childcare programmes more difficult. In a similar way, planning for the health needs of older members of society, most of whom are women, is difficult.

Gender-based violence provides an example of how the lack of statistics can impede gender mainstreaming in the health sector. Inadequate data affect the ability of the health sector to provide treatment and to collaborate effectively with other agencies, so that together they can provide a comprehensive service to women and also try to prevent recurrence of abuse. In many countries, statistics about violence against women are scanty, largely because of under-reporting. In the case of domestic violence, there is a tendency to keep it hidden within the family circle. The stigma attached to rape and the feeling that law enforcement officers may not treat it seriously lead to low reporting rates. Even when a woman seeks treatment in a hospital or clinic she may mask the real cause of her injuries. Health professionals, who may often have no specific training in recognising violence against women, remain

*'A Draft Framework for Designing National Policies with an Integrated Gender Perspective', paper prepared by Professor Lesley Doyal for the UN Expert Group Meeting on Women and Health, Mainstreaming the Gender Perspective into the Health Sector, Tunis, September 1998.

Gender-based violence provides an example of how the lack of statistics can impede gender mainstreaming in the health sector.

Traditionally, medical research has been male-dominated.

unsuspecting, even though the same woman presents repeatedly with extensive bruising, stating that she has yet again 'fallen down the stairs'.* In such cases, the health records will not indicate that treatment was necessitated by a gender-related problem. Thus, if a GMS in health is being introduced, it will start at a disadvantage if it intends to introduce special programmes for treating women with health problems arising form domestic violence or sexual abuse and rape.

Much can be done by governments to improve their data collection. They can use the UNDP gender indicators. Governments can, with assistance from international agencies, collect information which takes into account the health needs of both women and men. Meanwhile, health professionals' associations can accelerate the process by encouraging their members to record sex-disaggregated data and collect information about women's health which can then be fed into planning processes.

Male dominance of health research

Traditionally, medical research has been male-dominated. Unless it was concerned with conditions from which only women suffer, it has always been assumed that there is no difference in the health needs of women and men, with the result that women's special needs are ignored. Drug trials and other therapeutic and preventive measures have often involved only men. A major explanation put forward for this is the risk of damage to the foetus if the woman is pregnant. The result of this approach is that even though certain conditions, such as heart disease, depression and HIV/AIDS affect women and men differently, many of the relevant studies have been carried out exclusively on men. Women have therefore been treated with drugs which have been tested for safety and efficiency only on men. Yet it is known that drug dosages may affect women and men differently. Another consequence of this tendency to use only men in research studies is that there has been inequitable funding for conditions, such as breast cancer, that predominantly affect women.

*Nechas and D. Foley, *Unequal Treatment: What you don't know about how women are mistreated by the medical community*, New York, Simon and Schuster, 1994.

The US National Institute of Health (NIH), the largest government funding organ for medical research, spent only 13 per cent of its annual budget in the early 1990s on women's health. The five-year 'Physician's Health Study' on intake of aspirin and reduction of heart disease was carried out on 22,071 subjects, none of whom were women. A 20-year study on ageing involved only men, although women comprise the majority of the population over the age of 65. Most surprisingly, a project carried out by Rockefeller University on the impact of obesity on the tendency of women to develop breast cancer involved only men!

While the Beijing Platform for Action called on governments to ensure that research is both gender-sensitive and takes full account of the needs of women, much remains to be done to ensure that women's health is adequately addressed through the collection of sex-disaggregated data.

Most work in the health sector is carried out by women. They are, however, mostly to be found in the less well-paid and lower echelons of the health sector, whether as professionals or administrators. Most surgeons and physicians are men, while the most nurses, midwives or untrained health care providers are women. Even in countries where there are substantial numbers of women in medicine, they tend to be working as general practitioners, pediatricians or in community medicine, rather than as surgeons or in other highly specialised and better remunerated areas of medicine.

As far as decision-making is concerned, most permanent secretaries and chief medical officers, as well as those next in seniority, tend to be men. Unfortunately these senior men are unlikely to have received any training in gender awareness and may be unaware of the differences in the impact of health care on women and men.

... much remains to be done to ensure that women's health is adequately addressed through the collection of sex-disaggregated data.

Lack of gender perspective in medical education

The basic medical education provided in medical schools is overburdened with the technical aspects of curative medicine. Any attempt to introduce changes to the syllabus, including the incorporation of gender issues, is therefore fiercely resisted. Even courses on medical ethics are unlikely to include instruction in gender sensitivity and health professionals often have very little education about ethical principles such as respect for patients, the right to information, informed choice and confidentiality, all of which are critically important for ensuring that there is a gender perspective in patient treatment.

Fortunately, the need for continuing professional education has been increasingly accepted and this offers an excellent opportunity for providing education on gender issues to health professionals at all levels. So the gap which existed in their initial training can be remedied. In response to the need for such education, the CMA has developed continuing education modules that teach health professionals about compliance with ethical and human rights standards in the provision of health care. The materials focus on the obligations owed by health professionals to vulnerable and disadvantaged groups in the community. These groups include the majority of women in developing countries. The modules, which have been field-tested in a number of Commonwealth countries, include case studies on ethical and human rights violations involving women.

5. National Plans of Action for the GMS in Health: Commonwealth Examples

Participants at the Commonwealth workshops developed outline Plans of Action for the GMS in the health sector. It was understood that these were generic Plans of Action which should be adapted to national requirements in consultation with all stakeholders. They would then be adopted by governments as the GMS for their own health sector. Some examples of the Plans of Action are presented below.

Africa

This framework and Plan of Action was developed by participants from Botswana, Lesotho, Mozambique, Namibia, South Africa, Swaziland and Zimbabwe.

Vision

A health sector in which all women and men have equal rights and both are respected as equal partners at all levels of the health system. Within this framework, women and men will work in collaboration and partnership utilising their full potential to ensure that the specific health needs of all are adequately met. This is possible only where policies, programmes and procedures are gender sensitive. A prosperous society is envisaged, characterised by equal participation of women and men in the utilisation of health services at all levels.

Mission

To achieve gender equity and equality through strategic action such as:

- promoting political will;

- changing negative cultural values;

- strengthening partnerships among stakeholders;

- building capacity to introduce reform;

- promoting good professional practices in the provision of health for all.

Goal

To achieve the integration of gender into all national policies, programmes and activities which impact upon health.

Objectives
Policy and structural reform

- To establish a gender desk (appoint an officer and identify a structure);

- To provide health partners, i.e. service providers and other stakeholders with appropriate knowledge, skills and attitudes to ensure that there is gender sensitivity at all levels;

- To develop databases that are disaggregated by sex, age and location for use in planning and programme implementation;

- To include gender equality and equity in all policies, strategies and programmes;

- To create an enabling environment for effective implementation, monitoring and evaluation of gender integration in health policies and programmes;

- To strengthen essential national health systems research and the use of gender-sensitive research results in the formulation of health policies and programmes.

Recruitment and training

- To include gender and development in training on impact assessment in all ongoing education programmes;

- To use health professionals to facilitate partnership building among all stakeholders, including health ministries and all other ministries, NGOs and Intergovernmental Organisations to foster intra- and inter-sectoral networking;

- To support the use of gender equality and equity principles in the recruitment, training and promotion of health workers and encourage the use of these principles by providers and users of health services.

Specific programmes

- To increase resources for women's health including:
  - a) expanding women's access to appropriate health care
  - b) consolidating preventive health care for women
  - c) undertaking gender-sensitive initiatives towards reproductive health
  - d) reviewing and strengthening all reproductive health initiatives;

- To review and revise components of the health sector based on sex-disaggregated data in order to ensure accessibility of services;

- To publicise information about the health of women and men;

- To identify psycho-social problems that impinge on the health of women, men and children and develop programmes that meet these needs;

- To promote primary prevention of cancers of the cervix, uterus, breast, prostate and lungs;

- To review data available on malnutrition and address gender-related feeding practices and micro-nutrient deficiencies;

- To develop programmes that address the gender-based health needs of adolescents and the aged, and develop gender-sensitive programmes to address those needs;

- To formulate and implement gender-sensitive primary, secondary and tertiary preventive programmes to reduce diseases of affluence.

Strategies
Policies and structural reform

- Ratify international conventions relevant to women's rights and gender equality in health care;

- Establish a task force led by the Ministry of Health which will scrutinise all existing and new legislation for gender implications;

- Establish a committee of parliamentarians to support the

GMS and also seek support from Cabinet ministers and other executive councils;

- Include gender equality considerations in the core agenda of critical committees, for example the Cabinet;

- Conduct baseline surveys and organise a database with a gender perspective as a priority;

- Draft a document stating the principles for the introduction of gender issues in sectoral policies;

- Establish a Gender Desk and Gender Focal Point in the Ministry of Health and in Provincial Health Departments;

- Devise regular reporting mechanisms, for example an annual report on progress made in gender mainstreaming throughout the health system;

Recruitment, training and education

- Build capacity among all those involved in implementing the GMS in health by providing training in gender planning and analysis, and explaining the mechanisms and processes of the GMS. This will strengthen their ability to implement the GMS and promote the integration of gender issues into all development planning;

- Establish partnerships with stakeholders on specific programmes and sensitise them through workshops, media programmes, seminars, debates and advocacy;

- Mobilise and develop human, technical and financial resources which will support and plan priorities;

- Organise public awareness campaigns to promote the objectives of the GMS using the media, public consultations, etc.;

- Conduct training of trainers' workshops to develop expertise in gender integration;

- Organise training activities in gender awareness, gender planning and analysis for policy-makers, for example workshops, meetings and study tours;

- Improve methods of staff recruitment and conditions of service by taking gender equality and equity issues into consideration;

- Introduce training on the GMS and on gender mainstreaming in general in the pre-service and in-service training provided for all health personnel;

- Improve health education and school health programmes by including information on gender-based health problems;

- Review health training curricula to ensure that they incorporate gender issues;

- Improve training provided for traditional midwives in rural areas so that maternal morbidity and mortality rates can be reduced;

- Train male and female community workers in all aspects of reproductive health.

Specific programmes

- Establish mechanisms to review the practice of private and traditional medicine so that any activities which lead to poor quality care for women and children can be eliminated;

- Disseminate information on women's labour rights and on provisions to protect their occupational health;

- Monitor all health care delivery to ensure that it is gender sensitive;

- Increase coverage rates in mother and childcare in order to reduce mortality and morbidity rates through the services, focusing on:
  a) ante-natal care
  b) birth in institutions
  c) post-natal care
  d) family planning
  e) prevention of infectious diseases
  f) reducing malnutrition
  g) immunisation;
- Introduce education and counselling on family planning and complications in pregnancy and delivery, through activities such as regional workshops and community meetings;

- Ensure that women are involved in policy and programme development, taking care to involve vulnerable women such as those suffering from HIV/AIDS. In so doing women should work in partnership with men;

- Conduct surveys on abortion to obtain accurate and up-to-date information on the rate of incidence, predominant causes and complications experienced. On the basis of this data, establish practices which will minimise unplanned pregnancies and provide safe abortions where necessary;

- Introduce and strengthen communication channels between the Ministry of Health, and NGOs and the media by intensifying advocacy programmes and publishing periodic newsletters;

- Provide government subsidies for NGOs and women's organisations which organise programmes relevant to women's health;

- Incorporate gender sensitivity at all levels of education, including the use of gender-sensitive language in all educational materials;

- Strengthen programmes which address gender issues that have adverse effects on women's health, for example programmes dealing with:
  a) violence against women
  b) women and smoking
  c) women and alcohol
  d) women's high illiteracy rates.

Implementing agencies

The following list was drawn up of ministries and agencies which could be primary implementers of a GMS in health. The Ministry of Health would be the lead agency. However, the precise collaborating agencies would differ according to the actual situation in each country:

- Prime Minister/President and Cabinet;

- Members of Parliament and Party politicians;

- Ministry of Health staff;

- Staff from other participating ministries, for example Ministries of Finance, Planning, Women's/Gender Affairs, Social Services, Agriculture, Education and Justice;

- NGOs and trade unions;

- Community and religious organisations;

- Traditional leaders;

- Professional bodies;

- Intergovernmental organisations;

- The media.

Timeframes

- Initiatives to establish the GMS in health should commence immediately or as soon as possible if there are budgetary or long-term development plans which make immediate implementation difficult;

- The target for introducing sex-disaggregated data collection and increasing the percentage of women in senior decision-making positions was set at the year 2000;

- Most of the measures and activities considered necessary to carry out the strategies outlined above would continue indefinitely.

Resources

Human resources

Human resources required to ensure the effective implementation of the GMS would include the following:

- Political leaders;

- Officials in ministries and agencies to implement the GMS and provide necessary training;

- Gender focal points;

- Religious and traditional leaders;

- Evaluation teams.

Financial resources

Effective implementation of the GMS would involve reprioritisation of financial resources and merging of existing resources. This would involve:

- Health planners and providers;

- Health promoters and educators;

- Producers of gender-sensitive teaching, resource and promotional materials;

- Decisions about consultancies and consultancy fees;

- Provision of technological support;

- Decisions about the testing and use of drugs;

- Provision of transport for providers and users of health services.

Evaluation

The following examples were given of the types of indicators, which countries could use to evaluate progress in the implementation of the GMS.

Policy and structural reform

- National and gender equality policy adopted;

- Establishment of gender desk, task force, office;

- Approval of budget for gender desk, task force, office;

- Setting up of Gender Focal Points;

- Setting up of sex-disaggregated data collection processes;

- Development of gender-sensitive policies;

- Setting up of gender-sensitive health infrastructure in rural areas;

- Appropriate communication structures set up.

Qualitative measures

- International conventions relevant to women's rights and gender equality in health are ratified and implemented;

- Increased level of acceptance of principle of gender equality as verified by surveys, focus groups, etc.;

- Database on gender and health developed;

- Training of health personnel including senior personnel completed;

- New gender-sensitive terms of employment for employees and terms of reference for committees/task forces in place;

- Reporting mechanisms for gender and health issues in place, including efficient methods of dissemination;

- Publication of guidelines for mainstreaming gender into the health service;

- Establishment of a library/resource facility on gender and health;

- Information system on gender and health established;

- Reports on situational surveys on different health status of women and men completed and widely distributed;

- Greater gender sensitivity achieved in all health practices and programmes;

- More use made of health services by men;

- Increased use of gender planning and analytical skills by health care staff;

- Effectiveness of partnerships between all stakeholders working on gender and health issues at grassroots level.

Quantitative measures

- Number of human rights violations recorded;

- Number of gender-discriminatory laws repealed or revised;

- Number of health or health-related policies analysed for gender sensitivity;

- Number of additional professional staff appointed in specific gender-related areas of work;

- Number of women involved in process of policy and programme development up to the highest decision-making levels;

- Number of courses on gender equality organised for trainers and staff;

- Number of health curricula reviewed for coverage of gender and health issues and gender sensitivity;

- Number of reports on gender and health workshops, seminars, etc. distributed;

- Number of midwives trained;

- Degrees to which staff complement is gender-balanced, including at senior professional and administrative level;

- Increase in number of families accepting family planning;

- Number of men using health services;

- Number of deliveries attended by health professionals;

- Reduction in maternal and infant mortality rates and in complications during delivery;

- Increase in immunisation coverage;

- Reduction in cases of malnutrition;

- Increase in amount of research into gender and health issues and publication of results;

- Number of media programmes, articles, etc. available on gender and health issues;

- Availability of catalogue of newsletters, journals, etc. on gender and health issues;

- Number and coverage of social action programmes;

- Reports of community consultations and figures of attendance for women;

- Number of meetings with traditional leaders and distribution of reports.

Asia

The Plan of Action developed by participants from Malaysia is used as an example of plans of action developed at the Asia workshop.

Malaysian Plan of Action

Vision

- Healthy individuals, families and communities;

- A health system which is affordable, efficient, technologically appropriate, environmentally adaptable and consumer-friendly;

- A health system with an emphasis on quality, innovation, health promotion and respect for human dignity;

- A health system which promotes individual responsibility and community participation.

Objectives

- To ensure equitable sharing of resources, information, opportunities and benefits of development by women and men. Equity and justice should be the essence of development policies, which must be people-oriented so that women can contribute and realise their potential to the optimum.

- To integrate women in all sectors of development in accordance with their capabilities and needs; enhance quality of life for all; eradicate poverty, ignorance and illiteracy; and create a peaceful and prosperous nation.

Priorities in establishing a GMS in health

- Equity
- Good quality health care
- Accessibility of services
- Human resource development
- Good research facilities and reports
- Efficient health management information system.

Stakeholders

Government ministries and agencies
Ministry of Health
Ministry of Education
Ministry of Housing and Local Government
Other relevant ministries
Women's/Gender Affairs Division
Economic Planning Unit
Public Service Department
National Population and Family Development Board.

Private health sector
Private hospitals and clinics
Pharmaceutical industries
National Institute on Occupational Safety and Health.

Non-governmental organisations
Professional bodies
National Council of Women's Organisations
Consumer associations
Trade unions
Employer associations.

Outline of Plan of Action
The Action Plan should:

- Work within the existing structure, strengthening and redefining it and introducing gender equality principles;

- Develop new elements necessary for implementing the GMS.

Existing structures

1. Long-term plan (30 years)	Malaysian Vision 2020
2. Medium-Term Plan (10–20 years)	New Economic Policy: National Development Policy
3. Five-year Malaysia Development Plan and preparation of Eighth Plan	Review of 7th Malaysian Plan
4. Other plans and policies	Privatisation/health care financing, etc.

Figure 2. Existing National Machineries for the Advancement of Women in Malaysia

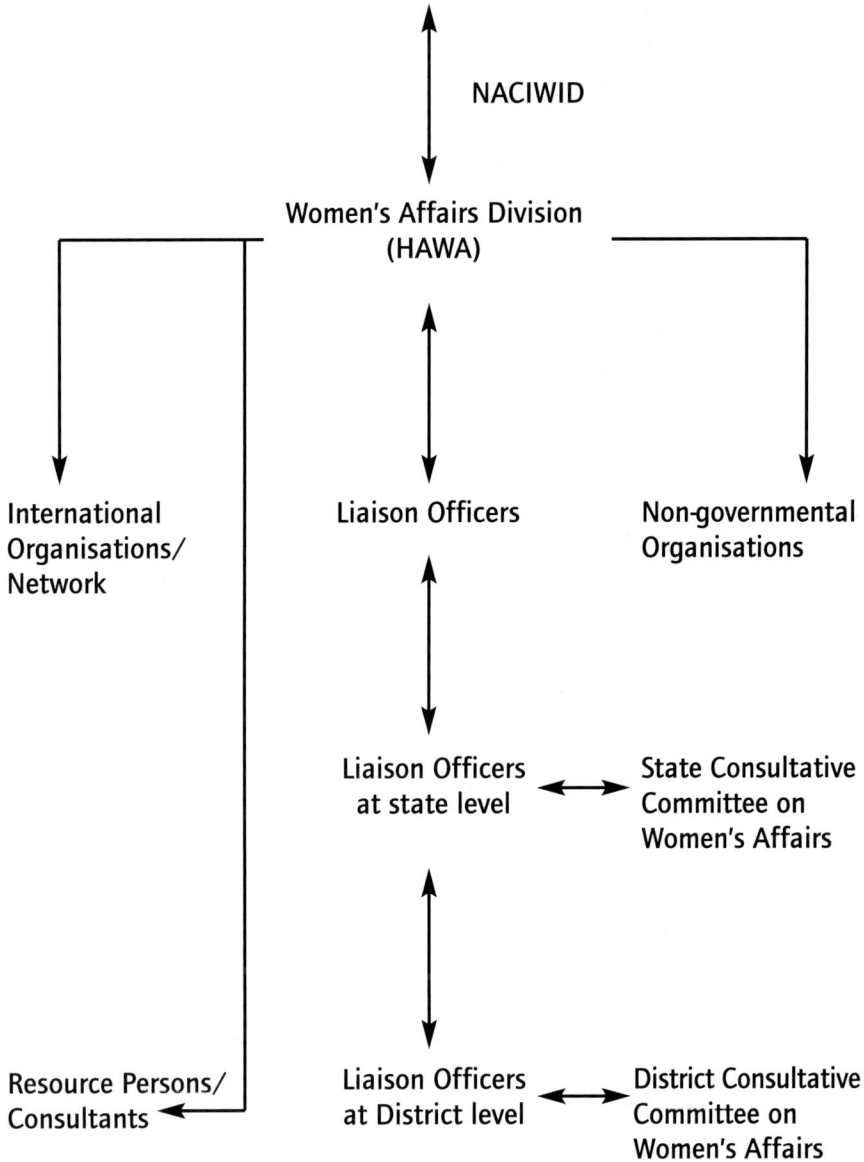

Table 3. Strategies for Implementing the GMS in Malaysia

Strategy	Activity	Stakeholders	Timeframe
Introducing gender-sensitive policies and programmes	Appraisal of existing policies for gender sensitivity	Economic Planning Unit, Women's Affairs Department	5-yearly
	Gender analysis of Ministry of Health Programmes, curricula and services	Ministry of Health	Mid-term (review every two and a half years)
	Development of GMS indicators	Commonwealth Secretariat	
Organising training	Management training, programmes leading to increased promotion opportunities for women	Women's Affairs Division	Ongoing
	Training of trainers on gender awareness, gender analysis and planning, etc.	University Medical Schools	
	Integrating gender into all types of curriculum development	Malaysian Medical Association	
	Gender sensitisation training for all health workers	Commonwealth Secretariat, WHO, Women's NGOs	
Improving communication on gender integration	Dissemination of materials on gender and health	Ministries of Information and Education	Ongoing
	Setting up efficient intersectoral communication mechanisms	Ministry of National Unity and Development	
Securing resources for GMS	Organising adequate and appropriate human deployment	Economic Planning Unit	Yearly
	Securing community resources for health-related activities	Ministry of Finance Public Services Department Ministry of Health	
Monitoring and evaluation	Use gender-sensitive indicators to monitor and evaluate implementation of GMS and its impact on clients and providers	Village committees, NGOs, Women's Affairs Department, Universities, Ministry of Health, Commonwealth Secretariat	Yearly

The Caribbean

The outline Plan of Action drawn up by participants from Barbados is used as an example of plans provided by participants from the Caribbean.

Barbados Plan of Action

Vision

The philosophy of the Government of Barbados is that health is a fundamental right. Good health does not exist simply because there is an absence of disease. Good health must enable people to lead spiritually, socially and economically productive lives where equity and equality prevail in a harmonious environment.

Mission

The mission of the Government of Barbados is to further strengthen the health sector to achieve gender equality and equity through the introduction of gender-sensitive policies and programmes. The health sector will work in collaboration with other sectors to enable individuals, families and communities to develop and adopt good health practices in order to achieve productive and healthy lifestyles.

Goal

The goal of the GMS in the health sector is to ensure the integration of gender into all government policies, programmes and activities which impact on health.

Objectives

- To review and evaluate existing systems, plans and structures to identify gender-based issues and problems;

- To make changes in the existing structures and develop new components so that a GMS can be established;

- To develop public education programmes on the GMS;

- To train all categories of staff in the health sector to be gender sensitive;

- To establish rapport with political parties; strengthen links between the Health Ministry and other Ministries; develop partnerships between the Ministry of Health and organisations involved in health care, for example NGOs, private sector organisations, trade unions, professional bodies and international agencies in order to promote gender mainstreaming in health;

- To build capacity in gender mainstreaming so that the goals of the GMS can be achieved;

- To promote the GMS by strengthening capacity to promote it;

- To ensure that all data collection and analysis is sex-disaggregated and use the data to plan and implement the GMS.

Stakeholder roles and responsibilities
Government policy-makers

- To formulate policies for the GMS;

- To allocate technical and financial resources to the GMS;

- To organise programmes to mobilise and educate the community;

- To establish institutional mechanisms for implementing the GMS;

- To set and monitor standards operative in the GMS implementation;

- To put in place a system for collating, analysing and disseminating all information on the GMS;

NGOs, professional bodies and community-based organisations

- To sensitise members and the public about gender mainstreaming and the GMS;

- To assist in the implementation of projects and programmes which are part of the GMS.

The media

- To sensitise and educate the public about the GMS.

Trade unions

- To provide information and advice on the GMS for Ministry of Health staff and trade union members in other collaborating ministries and organisations;

- To review their systems in the light of the gender mainstreaming approach and the gender equality and equity principles on which the GMS is based.

Table 4. Strategies for Implementing the GMS in Barbados

Issues	Strategic Goals	Targets	Measurement Evaluation	Institutional Mechanisms
Political will	To establish a GMS	Cabinet	Approval for the GMS	Ministries of Health and Education
Financial resources	To reallocate existing financial resources To access international funding	Finance officers Policy-makers	Funds allocated to GMS	Budgets of Ministries of Health, Education and international agencies
Training	To train trainers To sensitise health providers and relevant NGOs	Gender Focal Points, Heads of participating departments, Ministry of Health personnel	All Gender Focal Points, Ministry of Health personnel and Heads of participating departments trained	Training Divisions of Women's Bureau, Ministries of Health and Education
Human resources	To increase the staff at Women's Bureau	Women's Bureau	Increase in staff at Women's Bureau	Ministry of Labour and Community Development
	To identify Gender Focal Points in Ministry of Health and other participating ministries	Ministry of Health and other participating ministries	Gender Focal Points put in place	Ministries of Civil Service, Education and Health
Community support	To train NGOs and community-based organisations in the GMS	Management Executives of NGOs and organisations	Number of people trained on the GMS	University of West Indies Centre for Gender Studies, Centre for Continuing Studies, Institute of Social and Economic Research
Media: print and Electronic	To secure their partnership in the GMS	Editors, journalists	Level of reporting on GMS and gender issues	GMS Management Team, Government Information Service, Women's Media Watch, Men's Forum
Data collection	To establish a system for collecting sex-disaggregated data	All information systems	All records are disaggregated by sex	Data collection units

The South Pacific

Participants from Fiji produced the following outline of a Plan of Action for the GMS.

Vision

A health sector which provides equal rights and opportunities for women and men, with the overall goal of having a healthy and productive population.

Mission

The mission of the GMS in the health sector is to achieve gender equity and equality through appropriate strategic action.

Objectives

- To strengthen the enabling environment for gender main-streaming;

- To develop and strengthen health sectoral and system-wide commitment to gender mainstreaming;

- To strengthen the institutional capacity of the Ministry of Health to achieve gender mainstreaming in all health policies, programmes and services;

- To strengthen the institutional capacity of the Ministry of Women's Affairs to conduct advocacy for, and give advice on, gender mainstreaming;

- To encourage partnerships between the Ministry of Health and other ministries and organisations participating in the GMS;

- To incorporate gender training in national education and health training institutions.

Activities

- Implement international conventions and declarations which promote women's human rights and gender equality in health;

- Ensure that key stakeholders and central ministries (finance, national planning, public service commission) participate in the National Health Promotion Council;

- Appoint the National Health Promotion Council as the GMS Management Team;

- Link the GMS in Health Plan of Action with the national development plans;

- Arrange consultations between the Ministries of Finance, National Planning and Health on the integration of gender concerns into decision-making on national economic policies and budgetary processes;

- Integrate gender into all health policies and programmes through collaboration between the National Health Promotion Council and all ministries, IGOs, NGOs and organisations with programmes which impact on health;

- Strengthen the capacity of the planning unit of the Ministry of Health to produce gender-sensitive sectoral plans;

- Analyse public expenditure in the health sector and assess implications for the health of women, men, girls and boys, respectively;

- Develop indicators for measuring gender integration into the health sector;

- Conduct a periodic gender audit to assess responsiveness to gender concerns in the health sector;

- Establish a system to ensure that all data collected and analysed by the Ministry of health are disaggregated by sex and age;

- Organise gender training for all levels of health workers (including policy-makers and senior administrators) in all participating ministries and organisations.

References

1. *Gender Planning and Development: Theory, Practice and Training*, 1995, New York and London: Routledge.

2. Reports of Commonwealth workshops on Gender Management Systems in the Health Sector:
   Cape Town, South Africa   1996
   Colombo, Sri Lanka   1997
   Port of Spain, Trinidad   1998
   Fiji   1998
   Basseterre, St Kitts and Nevis   1999
   Halifax, Canada   1999
   Entebbe, Uganda   2000
   Nicosia, Cyprus   2001

3. *Gender Management Systems Handbook*, Commonwealth Secretariat, 1999

4. *A Draft Framework* (see p. 49)